REMINISCING
OUR HERITAGE

The 70s to the Millennium

DANNY WALSH

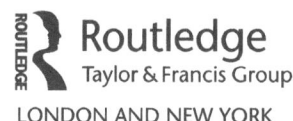

Routledge
Taylor & Francis Group

LONDON AND NEW YORK

First published 2014 by Speechmark Publishing Ltd.

Published 2017 by Routledge
4 Park Square, Milton Park, Abingdon, Oxon OX14 4RN
605 Third Avenue, New York, NY 10017

Routledge is an imprint of the Taylor & Francis Group, an informa business

Design and artwork by Moo Creative (Luton)

British Library Cataloguing in Publication Data
A catalogue record for this book is available from the British Library

ISBN 13: 978-0-86388-989-9 (pbk)

CONTENTS

Introduction

This book is designed to be used by anybody working with older adults in residential, nursing and day care facilities. It provides a wealth of reminiscence material which can be used in a number of ways to rekindle memories and provide stimulating activities such as quizzes and discussion. The sharing of memories is a very therapeutic tool, allowing people to feel a sense of belonging to their generation. It is of special value when working with those living with dementia as it helps them to retain a sense of who they are and their own unique history. Knowing about the individual you are caring for is a key aspect of providing good care, and using reminiscence gives carers the opportunity to gain that insight and so make meaningful connections with the person.

Each year covered in the book is divided into the sections 'Major events', 'On the home front', 'Music', 'Television', 'Screen and page', 'Sport' and 'Do you remember?' Many sections can be easily turned into quizzes and it would be simple to form a quiz from each year's material. One cannot cover all that happened in these years nor highlight all the associations each event or fact triggers, so the material is intended to be expanded on by the memories it triggers in clients during discussion. So, for example, where a film title is mentioned, ask if people can recall the stars of the film, its plot and how it ended. The 'Major events' section will trigger lots of opinions too, as it covers the political events of the decades, so try to get the client groups to discuss the ethical and moral dilemmas these posed at the time. Try also to get people to relate the past to the modern world and reflect on the progress made, and whether that progress is always such a good thing! The sections 'On the home front' and 'Do you remember?' are intended to reflect more of the ordinary events that are closest to most of our lives, such as having to go shopping and wash up. These are rich reminiscence areas to explore as we all share these experiences. The book is intended for use with individuals and groups, but you will discover that in a group one person's memories will trigger another's and so what seems like a small topic can last for the whole session as we all try to tell our personal tales.

While the content has a UK bias, it also covers the major world events of the decades. I have included a blank page for each year for you to record your own personal landmarks and achievements and also those of your local town or community. These personal and local events are the key to our individuality and as care workers we need to heed the importance of connecting with these important and personal events in our clients' lives.

1970

Major events

January

In the UK the half-crown or 'two and six' (12.5p today) ceased to be legal tender and the age of majority was reduced from 21 to 18.

The first Boeing 747 or 'Jumbo Jet' landed at Heathrow airport. The Pan Am flight had taken off from New York and gave impetus to the growing popularity of foreign holidays.

March

Rhodesia declared itself a republic, severing its ties with the UK and calling itself Zimbabwe.

May

Four students were killed by National Guardsmen at Kent State University, Ohio. They were protesting against the USA sending troops to Cambodia.

The Beatles release their final album, *Let It Be.*

The England cricket team's South African tour was called off due to anti-apartheid protests.

England football captain Bobby Moore was arrested in Bogata, Columbia on suspicion of stealing a bracelet.

June

The Conservative Party leader Ted Heath was surprisingly elected as Prime Minister after defeating the Labour Party led by Harold Wilson, who had been well ahead in the polls. This represented a huge swing to the Tories. It was also the first time that 18-year-olds had been allowed to vote. Heath was a keen yachtsman and many suspected that he would rather have been aboard his yacht *Morning Cloud* than in Parliament. He later made Margaret Thatcher his Education Secretary.

The 'Troubles' were still flaring in Northern Ireland with riots following the arrest of Ulster MP Bernadette Devlin.

July

The adventurer Thor Heyerdahl crossed the Atlantic from Morocco to Barbados in a papyrus boat, *Ra II*. It took 57 days.

A national dock workers' strike stopped imports and exports and the troops were put on standby.

September

Three planes hijacked by Palestinian terrorists were blown up in Jordan. They held the passengers hostage until seven detained Palestinians were released.

The 'binmen' went on strike, causing bags of rubbish to pile up in the streets.

November

Charles de Gaulle, ex-President of France, died.

December

The Beatles officially disbanded as Paul McCartney brought a lawsuit to dissolve the group.

Also this year ... computer floppy disks were developed and large oilfields were discovered in the North Sea. This year also saw the ten-shilling note go out of circulation.

On the home front

Life expectancy in 1970 was around 69 years for men and 75 for women. Nearly half of all households didn't have use of a car and the largest part of household expenditure went on food and soft drinks. Colour television was still in its infancy; the average home cost around £5,000 and a Mini car about £600. Washday was easier now, with around 65 per cent of households having a washing machine. For many poorer households, however, the trip to the launderette was still obligatory.

The must-have toy of the year was the Raleigh Chopper bicycle at a cost of £32. Sounds cheap today, but this was the average weekly wage at the time! The Chopper designer also gave us the bright orange Reliant Bond Bug. The Stylophone was another popular toy. The arrival of Jumbo Jets increased the popularity of foreign holidays with more

Routledge
Taylor & Francis Group

people taking advantage of the boom in package deals. Benidorm, Torremolinos and the various Costas in Spain were popular destinations, giving people a heady mix of sunshine, paella and sangria. Holiday camps such as Butlins and Pontins were still popular but their appeal was to dwindle over the decade. Holidays abroad were educating our palates and in the kitchen labour was saved with the rise of ready meals such as Vesta curries and Chinese dishes which just had to be rehydrated in the saucepan. These helped to make television dinners popular.

In the world of fashion, hot pants were all the rage. These were often quite revealing and didn't suit everyone. It soon became apparent that not all who wore them had checked in the mirror first! For boys, 'Tuff' Wayfinder shoes had imprints of the moon's surface on the soles which left an imprint of it on the ground … not as good as the mid-1960s versions with the animal tracks on the soles and the compass in the heel! From November the *Sun* newspaper featured a topless model on page 3, perhaps indicating a broadening of minds yet acknowledging too that sexism was alive and well in the early 1970s.

Music

The 1970s was an era of festivals. Following 1969's Woodstock came the second Isle of Wight festival with The Who, The Jimi Hendrix Experience, Melanie, and Richie Havens, to name but a few. The entry fee was just £3! 1970 also saw the first Glastonbury festival take place and Irish singer Dana won the Eurovision Song Contest with *All Kinds of Everything*. Sadly both Janis Joplin and Jimi Hendrix died this year from drug incidents, both aged 27. Can you recall who sang these popular 1970 singles?

In the Summertime	Mungo Jerry
Bridge Over Troubled Water	Simon and Garfunkel
All Right Now	Free
Band of Gold	Freda Payne
Big Yellow Taxi	Joni Mitchell
Can't Help Falling in Love	Andy Williams
Cracklin' Rosie	Neil Diamond

Routledge
Taylor & Francis Group

Knock Three Times	Tony Orlando and Dawn
Lola	The Kinks
Tears of a Clown	Smokey Robinson and the Miracles
Voodoo Child	Jimi Hendrix Experience
Spirit in the Sky	Norman Greenbaum
Wand'rin' Star	Lee Marvin
You Can Get It If You Really Want	Desmond Decker

The Rock opera *Jesus Christ Superstar* was among many memorable albums. See if you can remember the artist from the LP title:

Moondance	Van Morrison
Sweet Baby James	James Taylor
Band of Gypsies	Jimi Hendrix
Candles in the Rain	Melanie
Let It Be	The Beatles
Live at Leeds	The Who
In Rock	Deep Purple
After the Goldrush	Neil Young
Close to You	The Carpenters
Mad Dogs and Englishmen	Joe Cocker
All Things Must Pass	George Harrison

Ɽ Routledge
Taylor & Francis Group

Television

The comedy *On the Buses* was at the height of its popularity. It starred
Reg Varney as bus driver Stan Butler and Stephen Lewis played the
grumpy inspector Blakey whose catchphrase was 'I 'ate you, Butler'. First
shown in 1969, *Star Trek* was well on the way to becoming a cult television series, going
'where no man has gone before'! Travelling in the *Starship Enterprise* were William
Shatner as Captain Kirk and Leonard Nimoy as Spock. Staying in space, *Dr Who* was
being played by Jon Pertwee, who had taken over from Patrick Troughton. It was the first
time it was broadcast in colour. Old favourite *Coronation Street* was 10 years old.

New television programmes this year included *A Question of Sport* hosted by David Vine
with rugby player Cliff Morgan and boxer Henry Cooper as team captains. The BBC's
drama series *Play for Today* began a 14-year run. It was responsible for many fine
dramas from gritty political snapshots to the darkly comic. Standout plays included
Abigail's Party, *Spend, Spend, Spend* and *Edna the Inebriate Woman* starring
Patricia Hayes. The comedy series *The Goodies* also began this year with Graeme Garden,
Tim Brooke-Taylor and Bill Oddie.

Many older programmes were still very popular: can you remember their stars and
presenters in 1970?

Dixon of Dock Green	Jack Warner ('Evening all'!)
Opportunity Knocks	Hughie Green
Crackerjack	Michael Aspel
The Sky at Night	Sir Patrick Moore
Blue Peter	John Noakes, Peter Purves and Valerie Singleton
Grandstand	Frank Bough
Animal Magic	Johnny Morris
Play School	Brian Cant
It's a Knockout	David Vine with Eddie Waring as referee
The Golden Shot	Bob Monkhouse with Ann Aston and Bernie the Bolt!

Dad's Army	Arthur Lowe, Captain Mainwaring
	John Le Mesurier, Sergeant Wilson
	Clive Dunn, Lance-Corporal Jones
	John Laurie, Private Frazer

The other main characters were Pike, Godfrey, Walker and ARP Warden Hodges.

Screen and page

The film M.A.S.H., about an army field hospital in the Korean War, starred Donald Sutherland as Hawkeye and Elliot Gould in the title roles, with other characters such as Radar, Major Frank Burns and Hot Lips Houlihan. One major British film was the story of a young boy and his pet falcon called *Kes*.

Can you name the stars of these other popular 1970 films?

Paint Your Wagon	Lee Marvin
Ryan's Daughter	Sarah Miles, Robert Mitchum, John Mills
Airport	Burt Lancaster, Dean Martin
Butch Cassidy and the Sundance Kid	Paul Newman, Robert Redford
Catch 22	Alan Arkin

Also released this year in the USA was Disney's *Aristocats*.

In literature, the year's important books included Germaine Greer's international feminist bestseller *The Female Eunuch*, Ted Hughes' dark and mythological book of poetry *Crow*, Roald Dahl's children's tale of foxes versus farmers *Fantastic Mr Fox* and Richard Bach's philosophical story of an outcast bird *Jonathan Livingston Seagull*.

Routledge
Taylor & Francis Group

Sport

In football, Martin Peters became the UK's first £200,000 footballer on transferring from West Ham to Spurs. England were knocked out of the Mexico World Cup in the quarter-finals by, guess who, West Germany. Brazil won the final (the Jules Rimet trophy) for the third time and were thus allowed to keep it. The must-have souvenirs for boys were the silver coins of the England squad you got when you filled your car up with Esso petrol. Can you also remember the England Squad's World Cup song *Back Home*?

In golf, Britain's Tony Jacklin won the US Open and in racing Nijinsky became the first horse for 35 years to win the English Triple Crown with wins in the Epsom Derby, the St Leger and the 2000 Guineas.

Do you remember?

On the sweet front, can you recall bubble gum in flat packs with collecting cards? Popular series were the World Cup, Star Trek, the Bionic Woman and the Million Dollar Man. Late 1960s versions included Batman and Robin and The Man from U.N.C.L.E. When you had the whole set you could arrange the backs to produce a poster. Another popular treat was the Curly Wurly as advertised by Terry Scott dressed as a schoolboy. Can you also recall free toys in cereal packets and cardboard cut-out wild animal heads on the backs of the cereal boxes? As a consequence of the bubble gum and toffee, can you also recall having gas at the dentist before the invention of nerve-numbing injections?

1970 Personal and local events

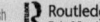

Routledge
Taylor & Francis Group

1971

Major events

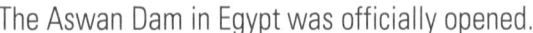

January

Divorce law reforms allowed couples to divorce after two years' separation and introduced the grounds of irretrievable breakdown.

The Aswan Dam in Egypt was officially opened.

The first ever UK postal workers' strike occurred, led by trade unionist Tom Jackson. It lasted 47 days. The workers were pursuing a 19.5 per cent pay rise. In the same year the Queen's allowance was raised by over 50 per cent.

Idi Amin seized power in Uganda and proclaimed himself president.

February

Decimal currency was introduced on the 15th. It was known as D-Day as people had to begin to think in 'p's instead of 'd's (old pence). A new shilling was 5p instead of 12d! Can you remember that there were 20 shillings in a pound and 12d in a shilling?

May

The *Daily Sketch*, Britain's oldest tabloid, ceased publication and was absorbed into the *Daily Mail*. It cost 2p!

July

Apollo 15 was launched. Its astronauts made three trips in the moon buggy *Lunar Rover*.

Clydeside shipbuilders took control of the Glasgow shipyards with a 'work in'.

August

George Harrison staged the Concert for Bangladesh in New York in aid of flood and civil war victims.

The UK government brought back internment without trial for terrorists and rounded up many IRA suspects.

 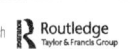 Routledge
Taylor & Francis Group

9

Chay Blyth becomes the first person to sail non-stop around the world from east to west (against the wind). It took him 292 days!

October
Walt Disney World opened in Florida.

An IRA bomb exploded at the top of the Post Office Tower in London.

November
The first commercial microprocessor became available.

December
An Ulster Volunteer Force bomb killed 15 people in a Belfast bar.

East Pakistan became independent Bangladesh after a bloody struggle.

Also this year ... the population of Britain was around 54 million. Several key inventions were made, such as the digital watch and the pocket calculator, which was useful for trying to work out how much things were in the new decimal currency. There were still troubles and suffering in Bangladesh and Northern Ireland, and major protests in the USA against the Vietnam War.

On the home front

Petrol was the equivalent of 7p a litre and the average salary was around £2,000. Other goods sound similarly cheap, with milk at 6p a pint, a Mars bar 2p, a first-class letter 3p and the price of a ticket to see the FA Cup final was £2. A trip to the cinema would only set you back about 30p. Fewer people had cars and most people did not use a credit card. About 90 per cent of households had a television, although most were still black and white.

The Morris Marina replaced the Morris Minor, which had been produced for 23 years. You still see Morris Minors lovingly tended, but few would recognise the Marina.

In toys, the craze was for Klackers – two plastic balls on a string which were banged together very quickly. They caused many an injury and were banned in many schools. Another early 1970s craze was the bright orange Space Hopper. It was a large rubber ball with a smiley face and handles which you sat on and bounced around. In fashion, platform shoes with thick soles were all the rage and were worn by many to make them look taller. Men's shirts were also getting wide, droopy collars and trousers were nearly all flared and often in bright colours. Check patterned Oxford bags were also popular. A throwback to the 1940s, these were extra wide with turnups. In tartan they were soon to be adopted by the Bay City Rollers.

School playground games still included British Bulldog, which led to many grazes and bruises as you tried to avoid getting caught. Marbles and conkers were still played but football was as popular as ever, with goalposts made from school jumpers and jackets thrown on the ground. Boys were forever getting told off for tearing the knees out of their trousers.

No party in 1970 was complete without a 'party four' or 'party seven' can of draught beer. These were nigh-on impossible to open without showering everyone with warm beer. Better to stick with wine at an average of £1 a bottle. A pint in the pub would set you back around four shillings or 20p, about the same as a packet of 20 cigarettes. A loaf of bread cost around 9p and home baking was much more prevalent than it is today. The Homepride flour advertising character Fred was very popular, with many homes having 'Fred' flour shakers or salt and pepper pots somewhere in the kitchen. Their advertising message was 'Graded grains make finer flour'.

Music

Many classic albums such as *Who's Next* were released this year, so see if you can guess the artist from the LP title.

Untitled/Four Symbols	Led Zeppelin
Tapestry	Carole King
Electric Warrior	T. Rex
Paranoid	Black Sabbath
Sticky Fingers	The Rolling Stones
Ram	Paul McCartney
Tarkus	Emerson, Lake and Palmer
Fireball	Deep Purple
Imagine	John Lennon

Routledge
Taylor & Francis Group

Hunky Dory	David Bowie
Fog on the Tyne	Lindisfarne

The singles charts similarly had a wealth of good songs, which started to reflect less of a Rock music emphasis.

Your Song	Elton John
Knock Three Times	Dawn
Maggie May	Rod Stewart
Get It On	T. Rex
Rose Garden	Lynn Anderson
It's Impossible	Perry Como
Brown Sugar	The Rolling Stones
Chirpy Chirpy Cheep Cheep	Middle of the Road
Indiana Wants Me	R. Dean Taylor
You've Got a Friend	James Taylor
Stoned Love	The Supremes
I'll Be There	The Jackson Five
Grandad	Clive Dunn
My Sweet Lord	George Harrison
I Hear You Knocking	Dave Edmunds
Gypsies, Tramps and Thieves	Cher
When I'm Dead and Gone	McGuinness Flint
Sweet Caroline	Neil Diamond
Tokoloshe Man	John Kongas

The Christmas number one was Benny Hill's *Ernie (The Fastest Milkman In The West)*.

Cult Rock musician Jim Morrison died this year aged 27, as did jazz legend Louis 'Satchmo' Armstrong aged 71.

Television

In January Open University broadcasts began. In *Coronation Street* Valerie Barlow was electrocuted by a faulty hairdryer and died in the ensuing fire. A drama series called *Elizabeth R* starring Glenda Jackson was popular and the first *Two Ronnies* was shown.

Programmes which debuted this year included *Upstairs Downstairs*, *Parkinson*, *The Onedin Line*, *The Old Grey Whistle Test* and *The Comedians*. The comedians included Frank Carson, Charlie Williams and Bernard Manning. The comedy show *Monty Python's Flying Circus* was very popular: its famous sketches included Dead Parrot, Spanish Inquisition, Nudge Nudge and The Ministry of Silly Walks. *The Generation Game* presented by Bruce Forsyth was also popular with its silly games, conveyor belt and 'cuddly toy' … 'Didn't she do well!' By the end of this year all television was broadcast in colour, although many people still only had black and white sets.

Many older programmes were still very popular. Can you remember some of their stars and presenters in 1971?

Monty Python's Flying Circus	Graham Chapman, John Cleese, Eric Idle, Michael Palin, Terry Gilliam, Terry Jones
Steptoe and Son	Wilfrid Brambell, Harry H. Corbett
Call My Bluff	Robert Robinson, Frank Muir, Patrick Campbell
Please Sir!	John Alderton
Magpie	Susan Stranks
All Gas and Gaiters	Derek Nimmo
Crossroads	Noele Gordon

The Galloping Gourmet was a popular cookery show presented by Graham Kerr. He was famous for drinking copious amounts of wine while cooking.

Routledge
Taylor & Francis Group

Screen and page

Get Carter starring Michael Caine premiered this year in Los Angeles and the seventh James Bond film *Diamonds are Forever* was released. Shirley Bassey sang the title song and Sean Connery played Bond, but can you name the stars of these other popular 1971films?

Dirty Harry	Clint Eastwood
The French Connection	Gene Hackman
The Godfather	Marlon Brando
Death in Venice	Dirk Bogarde
Love Story	Ali MacGraw, Ryan O'Neal
Fiddler on the Roof	Topol
A Clockwork Orange	Malcolm McDowell
Walkabout	Jenny Agutter
Straw Dogs	Dustin Hoffman
Bedknobs and Broomsticks	Angela Lansbury
Sunday Bloody Sunday	Peter Finch, Glenda Jackson

In literature, Roger Hargreaves' *Mr Men* children's books were first published. Can you remember the authors of these other books?

The Day of the Jackal	Frederick Forsyth
Adolf Hitler: My Part in His Downfall	Spike Milligan
The Moon's a Balloon	David Niven
Riotous Assembly	Tom Sharpe
Briefing for a Descent into Hell	Doris Lessing

Routledge
Taylor & Francis Group

Sport

Arsenal became only the second club this century to win the double, winning the First Division and the FA Cup by beating Liverpool 2–1 with a late goal from Charlie George. In cricket, the first ever one-day international was played between Australia and England in Melbourne, with Australia winning by five wickets. Can you answer these other 1971 sporting questions?

Arsenal's captain   *Frank Mclintock*

Inter-Cities Fairs Cup winners   *Leeds United*

Where did a crush kill 66 football fans on 2 January?   *Ibrox Park*

Which Scot won the Monaco Grand Prix?   *Jackie Stewart*

Who captained the British team to victory in the Admiral's Cup yacht race?
Prime Minister Edward Heath

Who was stripped of a show jumping victory for giving a V sign?   *Harvey Smith*

Who beat Muhammad Ali in the 'Fight of the century'?   *(Smokin') Joe Frazier*

Which golfer won the US Open, Canadian Open and British Open?   *Lee Trevino*

Which horse won the Epsom Derby, the King George VI and Queen Elizabeth Stakes at Ascot and the Prix de l'Arc de Triomphe?   *Mill Reef*

Which Australian won the women's singles at Wimbledon?   *Evonne Goolagong*

Do you remember?

Dansette mono record players in wooden boxes with lift-up lids and stacking 10 singles up at a time!

The floppy disks with snippets of pop songs on given away by teenage magazines!

Uri Geller and his spoon-bending antics!

Evel Knievel setting a world record by jumping 19 cars on his Harley-Davidson!

The boxer Henry Cooper urging us to 'Splash it all over'… Brut deodorant, that is!

1971 Personal and local events

Routledge
Taylor & Francis Group

1972

Major events

January

French singer Maurice Chevalier died; his songs included *Thank Heaven for Little Girls.*

A national miners' strike began (their first since 1926). It was to make the government declare a state of emergency and stopped coal getting to the power stations, triggering major power cuts.

The liner *Queen Elizabeth* was destroyed by fire in Hong Kong.

Prime Minister Edward Heath signed Britain into the Common Market in Brussels. Unemployment had doubled since Heath came to power two years previously and stood at over a million for the first time since the 1930s.

January 30 became known as 'Bloody Sunday' as 13 Catholics were shot by troops breaking up a demonstration in Londonderry. Meanwhile the IRA were running their own justice campaign, tarring and feathering any girls caught fraternising with British troops.

February

The first Winter Olympics to be held in Asia were opened in Tokyo but there were no medals for the Brits!

President Nixon became the first US president to visit China, where he held talks with Chairman Mao Tse-tung.

The IRA bombed Aldershot barracks, killing six people. Earlier this month the British Embassy in Dublin had been burnt down.

March

The last trolley bus system in the UK closed in Bradford.

An exhibition of the treasures of Tutankhamun's tomb opened at the British Museum.

The UK imposed direct rule in Northern Ireland.

May

Israeli commandos rescued 92 hijack victims at Entebbe airport, Uganda.

Actress Margaret Rutherford died. She starred on the London stage and later made a successful film career with such gems as *Passport to Pimlico* and *The VIPs*. She also starred as Miss Marple in many Agatha Christie films such as *Murder Most Foul*.

The 'Spaghetti Junction' motorway interchange was opened, completing the motorway link between London and the Scottish border, 300 miles away.

The Duke of Windsor, former British monarch, died in Paris. He had abdicated 35 years previously to marry the American divorcee Wallis Simpson.

July

The first official Gay Pride march was held in London.

In Belfast 22 bombs exploded, killing 13 and wounding 130.

Dock workers went on strike.

August

Idi Amin expelled 50,000 British Asians from Uganda, accusing them of sabotaging the Ugandan economy; they began arriving in the UK in September.

September

The school leaving age was raised to 16 in England and Wales.

Terrorists attacked the Israeli building at the Munich Olympics. Eleven of the athletics team were killed.

Two trawlers were sunk by an Icelandic gunboat, triggering another 'Cod War'.

November

Prime Minister Heath announced a wage and prices freeze to fight inflation, while in the US President Nixon was re-elected. Also this month US forces mounted a heavy bombing campaign in Vietnam. The world was shocked by an iconic picture of naked children running away from the napalm bombing.

Routledge
Taylor & Francis Group

December

A devastating earthquake hit Nicaragua's capital Managua.

Also this year … three all-male Cambridge colleges began taking female undergraduates and we saw the advent of the personal computer. Many of us now wonder how we ever coped without one and without email!

On the home front

Cosmopolitan women's magazine arrived in the UK this year with a heady mixture of fashion, sex and celebrity. Also becoming popular was mail order shopping such as from Habitat. In fashion, designer labels were popular so that the discreet label tucked away inside an item of clothing became a loud message on the outside. People wanted to let others see that they had bought a fashionable or expensive label.

Television was dominating home life and in America the phrase 'couch potato' was coined in reference to the fact that many people spent their free time just lying on the sofa watching television and eating fast or junk food. Less and less fruit and vegetables were being eaten with the continuing rise of convenience foods such as readymade lasagne and fish fingers. By the end of the 1970s around half the population had freezers and people were developing the habit of doing a big weekly shop rather than topping up frequently at the local shops. The supermarkets were taking over and the local greengrocer was dying out. However, you still by and large got your milk delivered, and had to leave a cup out for the milkman to cover the bottle with to stop the bluetits pecking through and getting the cream!

Ford announced that its new top-of-the-range car, the Granada, would be built at Dagenham. Honda meanwhile began importing and selling its small hatchback, the Civic. But the top-selling car in the UK in 1972 was the Ford Cortina, which was now in its third model. It was cheap to run but prone to rust, so not many survive today.

Portable cassette players were becoming very popular, challenging the transistor radio, and the advent of compact cassettes allowed people to tape their LPs and singles and record from the radio to make their own compilations of their favourite songs.

Music

This was the age of the 'teeny bopper', with David Cassidy and The Osmonds. David Bowie released the album *The Rise and Fall of Ziggy Stardust and the Spiders from Mars*. Other classic albums included Andrew Lloyd Webber's *Jesus Christ Superstar*, *Harvest* by Neil Young and *Foxtrot* by Genesis.

The singles charts similarly had a wealth of good songs and some horrendous ones (you decide)! See if you can remember who had hits with these.

Could It Be Forever	David Cassidy
Puppy Love	Donny Osmond
Without You	Harry Nilsson
American Pie	Don McLean
School's Out	Alice Cooper
Long Haired Lover From Liverpool	Little Jimmy Osmond
Sylvia's Mother	Dr Hook
Rocket Man	Elton John
Sweet Talking Guy	The Chiffons
I'd Like To Teach The World To Sing	The New Seekers
I Can See Clearly Now	Johnny Nash
All The Young Dudes	Mott the Hoople
Hold Your Head Up	Argent
I Just Can't Help Believing	Elvis Presley
Lady Eleanor	Lindisfarne
Virginia Plain	Roxy Music
Layla	Derek and the Dominoes
Jeepster	T. Rex

Routledge
Taylor & Francis Group

Morning Has Broken	Cat Stevens
Heart of Gold	Neil Young

This year was also the year that the Moog synthesiser was patented. It was to become the backbone of much 1970s music.

Television

This year saw the pilot episode of *Are You Being Served?* with such characters as Mrs Slocombe, played by Mollie Sugden, Mr 'I'm free' Humphries, played by John Inman, and Frank Thornton as Captain Peacock. The quiz show *Mastermind*, hosted by Magnus Magnusson, began this year too, as did the less serious *Sale of the Century* with Nicholas Parsons. This year also saw the first episode of *Emmerdale Farm* and *Film 72* with Barry Norman.

On children's television, debuts included *Rainbow* with its characters Bungle and Zippy, *John Craven's Newsround* and *Record Breakers* with Roy Castle.

In *Coronation Street* the timid Emily Nugent finally married Ernest Bishop! However, many 1960s television shows were still popular, such as *Voyage to the Bottom of the Sea*, *Randall and Hopkirk (Deceased)*, *Man About the House* and *The Saint*. On Radio 4 the comedy panel game *I'm Sorry I Haven't a Clue* began, hosted by Humphrey Lyttelton and starring Graeme Garden, Bill Oddie and Tim Brooke-Taylor. On Radio 2 Terry Wogan began presenting the *Breakfast Show*.

Screen and page

Can you name the stars of these popular 1972 films?

The Godfather	Marlon Brando
Under Milk Wood	Richard Burton and Elizabeth Taylor
Sleuth	Michael Caine and Laurence Olivier
Frenzy	Barry Foster
Antony and Cleopatra	Charlton Heston and Hildegard Neil

Routledge Taylor & Francis Group

21

Deliverance	Burt Reynolds
The Poseidon Adventure	Gene Hackman, Shelley Winters and Ernest Borgnine
Cabaret	Liza Minnelli and Michael York

In the literary world, John Betjeman became Poet Laureate in October and this year's major publications included Seamus Heaney's *Wintering Out*, *The Odessa File* by Frederick Forsyth, *All Creatures Great and Small* by James Herriot and Richard Adams' *Watership Down*.

Two feminist magazines started this year, *Spare Rib* in the UK and *Ms* in the USA.

Sport

In football, Tottenham beat 'Wolves' 2–1 in the first ever EUFA Cup with two Martin Chivers goals. In Barcelona Scotland's Glasgow Rangers won the European cup, beating Dynamo Moscow 3–2. Can you remember the answers to these other 1972 sporting questions?

At the Olympic Games in Munich, which US swimmer won seven gold medals? *Mark Spitz*

From Belfast, who won the Olympic women's Pentathlon with a new world record? *Mary Peters*

Leeds United won the FA Cup for the first time, beating Arsenal 1–0 with an Allan Clark header. Who was their manager?   *Don Revie*

In the Football League, Derby County were winners for the first time under whose guidance?   *Brian Clough*

At the Olympics, which young (17) Soviet gymnast gave stunning performances, winning four gold medals?   *Olga Korbut*

Who won both the US Open and Wimbledon women's finals?   *Billie Jean King*

In golf, Jack Nicklaus won the US Open and the Masters, but who won the British Open? *Lee Trevino*

Routledge Taylor & Francis Group

Do you remember?

Hanging salted peanut dispensers with pictures of bikini-clad girls on!

Lava lamps and Andy Warhol-style pop art pictures and mirrors.

That suave television dandy with the moustache, played by Peter Wyngarde – Jason King.

Pick of the Pops hosted by Alan (Fluff) Freeman, which ended its long run this year. His catchphrases included 'Greetings, pop pickers' and 'not 'arf!' It had been a Saturday night must-listen for teenagers.

Routledge
Taylor & Francis Group

23

1972 Personal and local events

1973

Major events

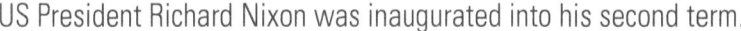

January

The UK entered the European Economic Community and a Union Jack was raised at the headquarters in Brussels.

US President Richard Nixon was inaugurated into his second term.

Prime Minister Heath introduced anti-inflation measures, prompting UK civil servants to go on strike for the first time.

March

Two IRA bombs went off in London, followed by two more five days later outside Whitehall and the Old Bailey, after a Northern Ireland referendum showed the majority who voted wanted to stay with the UK. Most Catholics did not vote.

The Queen opened the new London Bridge. The old one was sold and taken to Arizona!

Gifted writer and musical entertainer Noel Coward died aged 74.

April

VAT was introduced.

Artist Pablo Picasso died aged 91.

The very first hand-held mobile phone call was made this month in the USA.

May

The TUC (Trades Union Congress) called a one-day protest at the government's anti-inflation policy.

The 'Cod Wars' were in full swing, with the Navy sending three ships to protect British fishing vessels from Icelandic ships.

July

After an 11-year legal battle victims of the drug Thalidomide were finally paid compensation.

After June elections for the Northern Ireland power-sharing assembly, the first meeting was disrupted by a protest led by the Reverend Ian Paisley.

August

A fire at the modern Summerland holiday complex on the Isle of Man killed 50 holidaymakers.

September

General Pinochet and a military Junta took over Chile in a bloody coup.

A spate of IRA bombs targeted London.

October

Israel was attacked by Egypt and Syria on the religious holiday of the Day of Atonement or Yom Kippur. This Arab–Israeli War led to a worldwide oil shortage and soaring petrol prices.

The first independent, commercial local radio broadcasts began with the London Broadcasting Company.

Henry Kissinger was awarded the Nobel Peace Prize for his efforts to bring about a ceasefire in Vietnam.

November

The UK government took control of fuel distribution and declared a state of emergency due to the energy crisis caused by striking miners and electricians.

Princess Anne married Mark Phillips, a commoner, at Westminster Abbey. Around 500 million people worldwide watched on television and it was a national holiday in the UK.

December

John Paul Getty III, grandson of the American oil billionaire, was released after being kidnapped for ransom on 10 June. His mother had been sent his severed ear before the ransom of a million dollars was paid.

From midnight on the 31st a three-day week was introduced in the UK to combat coal shortages arising from industrial action and save electricity.

Routledge
Taylor & Francis Group

Also this year … The Irish 'Troubles' escalated, and by October interest rates were high and petrol prices were soaring.

On the home front

The first Pizza Hut opened in London this year and was an indication of the growing habit of eating out at fast food restaurants and of a broadening out of British tastes to embrace foreign foods. Things were also changing in the world of drinks cans as cans were being produced with 'push tabs' which you pressed into the tin with your thumb. These were soon to be replaced with the 'ring pull', thus making many a tin opener obsolete. Elsewhere disposable nappies were making life somewhat easier for mothers and almost every home had a Kodak Instamatic camera to capture those embarrassing holiday snaps.

In fashion, Mary Quant, who had taken credit for inventing and popularising the mini-skirt and hot pants, now added make-up to her range of merchandise. There was a plethora of similar products: for example, department store Biba launched its own range and Aqua Manda had a line aimed at teenagers with strong, orange, 'hippy', 'flower power' advertising themes and logos. For men there were Old Spice and Hai Karate aftershave and Cossack hairspray. These were usually advertised by male sports stars to try to overcome the embarrassed reluctance of the average male to use toiletries and 'perfumes'. Other fashion trends of the period were tank tops, often of a garish colour and pattern, and cheesecloth shirts. These were all the rage with both sexes.

Music

The classic Pink Floyd album *Dark Side of the Moon* was released this year, as were *Goodbye Yellow Brick Road* by Elton John, *Aladdin Sane* by David Bowie, *Tubular Bells* by Mike Oldfield, *Quadrophenia* by The Who, *Band on the Run* by Paul McCartney and Wings, and John Martyn's *Solid Air.*

The singles charts similarly had a wealth of 'memorable' songs:

Tie a Yellow Ribbon Round the Old Oak Tree	Dawn, featuring Tony Orlando
See My Baby Jive	Wizzard

 Routledge Taylor & Francis Group

Can the Can	Suzi Quatro
Rubber Bullets	10CC
Merry Xmas Everybody	Slade
The Jean Genie	David Bowie
Ballroom Blitz	The Sweet
You're So Vain	Carly Simon
Caroline	Status Quo
Whisky in the Jar	Thin Lizzy
Angie	The Rolling Stones
Wishing Well	Free
You Are the Sunshine of My Life	Stevie Wonder

Glam Rock was at its height and in contrast to the bleak political landscape it presented something of an antidote with its larger-than-life image. Dress was flamboyant, hair was coiffed and colourful, skin-tight sequined jumpsuits were all the rage, even for the boys, which helped to blur the gender divide, as did eye make-up and nail varnish.

Television

The television programme *Last of the Summer Wine* debuted this year. It was to run for 31 series until 2010. Its characters included Compo, Clegg and Nora Batty (played by Bill Owen, Peter Sallis and Kathy Staff). Also debuting was *Some Mothers Do 'Ave 'Em* with Michael Crawford, the talent show *New Faces* and *Whatever Happened to the Likely Lads?* This comedy was set in the North East and starred James Bolam and Rodney Bewes.

World of Sport at Saturday teatime was very popular, especially the wrestling commentated on by Kent Walton. Fans of 'grappling' tuned in by the million. Can you remember these heroes and villains? Big Daddy, Giant Haystacks, Mick McManus, Bert Royal, Vic Faulkner, Steve Logan, Jackie Pallo, Billy Two Rivers, Honey Boy Zimba and Pat Roach.

Routledge
Taylor & Francis Group

Coming to an end this year was the long-running successful comedy *Steptoe and Son* with Wilfrid Brambell and Harry H. Corbett. Also coming to the end after 20 years was *Watch with Mother*. This series of children's programmes had begun in 1953 and evolved with the years. Its favourites included *Andy Pandy*, *The Flower Pot Men*, *Rag, Tag and Bobtail*, *The Woodentops*, *Tales of the Riverbank*, *Camberwick Green* and *Fingerbobs*.

Screen and page

This year saw the release of *Live and Let Die* with Roger (the Saint) Moore playing Bond for the first time. In theatre the play *Equus* by Peter Shaffer opened. The British Rock and Roll film *That'll Be The Day* was released, starring David Essex and featuring Ringo Starr, Billy Fury and Keith Moon.

Can you name the stars of these other popular 1973 films?

Don't Look Now	Julie Christie and Donald Sutherland
Enter the Dragon	Bruce Lee
The Wicker Man	Edward Woodward, Christopher Lee and Britt Ekland
The Sting	Paul Newman and Robert Redford
The Exorcist	Linda Blair
Westworld	Yul Brynner
The Last Detail	Jack Nicholson

In literature, can you remember the authors of this year's top books?

The Ascent of Man	Jacob Bronowski
Awakenings	Oliver Sacks
The Honorary Consul	Graham Greene
Small is Beautiful	E. F. Schumacher
All Things Bright and Beautiful	James Herriot

This year also saw the death of one of our greatest poets, W. H. Auden. His poems included 'Funeral Blues', which later featured in the 1994 film *Four Weddings and a Funeral*.

Sport

This year saw England crash to cricket defeat against the West Indies. Captain Ray Illingworth commented that 'we were out-batted, out-bowled and out-fielded'. Gary Sobers was bowling for the 'Windies'.

In football, Liverpool won the Football League and Celtic were reigning in Scotland. Sunderland shocked Leeds United by beating them in the FA Cup Final. They were the first team outside the First Division to do this since the War. Jackie Charlton retired and his brother Bobby played his last game for Manchester United, and England goalkeeper Gordon Banks retired this year after losing his sight in one eye following a car crash.

Elsewhere, Jackie Stewart won the Formula One Drivers' Championship but pulled out of the last race and quit driving after a colleague was killed in practice. George Foreman beat Joe Frazier to become heavyweight champion of the world and Red Rum won the Grand National.

This year also saw the 'battle of the sexes' in tennis as the chauvinistic Bobby Riggs had declared that women were inferior to men at tennis. The women won with Billie Jean King defeating Bobby Riggs 6–4, 6–3, 6–3. It is still one of the most viewed tennis matches of all time.

Finally ... England, Scotland, Ireland, Wales and France *all* won the Five Nations Championship in Rugby Union! Each team ended with four points!

Do you remember?

This year Green Shield Stamps became Argos and sold goods for cash as well as stamps. Stamps were still issued well into the 1970s but largely at petrol stations. The stamps were originally a sort of loyalty scheme dating back to 1958. In 1973 you got one stamp for every 2½p you spent and the books soon filled up.

Can you also recall the GPO, which used to run the telephones? This Post Office Telecommunications Department was the predecessor to British Telecom. It used to run a favourite teenage service, 'Dial a Disc' (dial 16 or 160) and the 'Speaking Clock'!

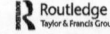

1973 Personal and local events

1974

Major events

January

New Year's Day was celebrated as a public holiday for the first time in the UK.

February

Author Alexander Solzhenitsyn was deported from the USSR after publication of his book *The Gulag Archipelago*, about his experiences in Soviet labour camps.

A general election was called because of the miners' strike, but it left no party with a majority. Tory leader Edward Heath tried to form a coalition with the Liberals but to no avail, and eventually resigned as Prime Minister; Harold Wilson and Labour stepped into power as a minority government.

March

The miners' strike ended when Labour offered a better pay deal. Twelve days after this 10 miners died in a methane gas explosion in Lancashire.

A state of emergency was declared in Northern Ireland and direct rule reimposed.

April

The Local Government Act created new counties of Humberside, Avon, West Midlands, Merseyside, Greater Manchester, Tyne and Wear, and South and West Yorkshire.

May

The right-wing National Front failed to win any council seats in London local elections but got 10 per cent of the vote.

June

An explosion ripped through a chemical plant at Flixborough, Lincolnshire, killing 28 and injuring 89. Two thousand houses were damaged and the village was evacuated as poisonous gas escaped.

Routledge
Taylor & Francis Group

Two IRA bombs went off at the Houses of Parliament and the Tower of London, injuring many people.

July

The Greek National Guard overthrew President Makarios in Cyprus, leading to Turkey invading to protect its communities. UN peacekeeping forces had to step in.

August

Richard Nixon became the first US President to resign, following the Watergate scandal. Vice-President Gerald Ford was sworn in as President.

October

MacDonald's opened its first restaurant in London.

The IRA bombing campaign intensified, with bombs in two pubs used by troops in Guildford. More London bombs were to follow, including one at a pub opposite a barracks in Woolwich and one in Oxford Street during the Christmas shopping period.

The UK's second general election this year gave Labour a narrow victory and saw Heath eventually lose the leadership of the Tory Party, to be replaced the following year by Margaret Thatcher. At the time inflation was running at 17.2 per cent, causing the costs of fuel and food to rise. Also on the rise was the Scottish National Party, which won 11 seats.

November

Lord Lucan disappeared after the murder of his children's nanny.

Two bombs exploded in central Birmingham pubs, killing 21 and injuring many more. The bombs were attributed to the IRA and six men were arrested. They were each given several life sentences.

The British government introduced the Prevention of Terrorism Act, outlawed the IRA and gave the police powers to detain suspected terrorists without trial.

December

Former Minister John Stonehouse was found living in Australia after having faked his own death. He was subsequently jailed.

Also this year … Chinese archaeologists discovered a 6,000-strong life-size terracotta army over 2,000 years old. They were lined up in battle formation and included horses and chariots. They were guarding the tomb of an emperor. And the skeleton 'Lucy' (*Australopithecus afarensis* to her friends) was discovered in Ethiopia. This early human ancestor lived around 3.9 million years ago. The world's first barcode scanner was introduced, and inflation was spiralling out of control across the globe as the recession deepened.

On the home front

The mid-1970s saw the height of 'teeny bopper' fashion and there were many teenage music magazines catering for this, such as *Pop Swap*, *Disco 45* and *Look In.* Other popular music papers included *Sounds*, *New Musical Express* and *Melody Maker.*

Marketing was becoming increasingly clever and humorous, and it was in 1974 that Cadbury's introduced alien robots advertising Smash instant potato. The robots couldn't stop laughing at the way we 'earthlings' peel, slice and then boil our potatoes before smashing them all to pieces. Instant puddings were fashionable too: Angel Delight and Instant Whip were favourites, with butterscotch a popular flavour. This year also saw the first domestic microwave cooker sold in the UK, heralding a boom in ready meals over the next few years as the fashion for microwave cookery caught on.

Indian restaurants and pizzas were becoming increasingly popular and Delia Smith rose to fame with her cookery show *Family Fare.* Dinner parties were still fashionable and hostess trolleys and soda siphons were the accessories to such events, which were often more like informal disco parties. There was often no set meal, just a help-yourself buffet with a selection of sweet and savoury items. The basic mix was plenty of flavoured crisps, cheese with pineapple on cocktail sticks, cheese straws, cocktail sausages, quiche, celery sticks, prawn cocktails and vol au vents. On the sweet side Walnut Whips went down well and to drink, the sweet German Rieslings such as Blue Nun were in vogue, as were Mateus Rosé, Cinzano, and 'anytime, anyplace, anywhere, it's the bright one, it's the light one, it's … Martini. Bottles of Chianti in wicker baskets were popular too, perhaps as a way of showing people that you had been abroad to Spain for your package holiday.

Music

The Eurovision Song Contest from Brighton, hosted by Katie Boyle, saw Swedish group Abba shoot to stardom after winning with *Waterloo*. This year was the height of 'Rollermania', with the tartan-clad Bay City Rollers having hits with *Bye Bye Baby* and *Give a Little Love*. Other number ones were:

Tiger Feet	Mud
When Will I See You Again?	The Three Degrees
Kung Fu Fighting	Carl Douglas
Seasons In The Sun	Terry Jacks
Annie's Song	John Denver
You're the First, the Last, My Everything	Barry White
I Shot the Sheriff	Eric Clapton
Gonna Make You a Star	David Essex
Devil Gate Drive	Suzi Quatro

Television

Kojak came to our small screens with Telly Savalas as the lollipop-sucking detective. Three popular comedies also began. *It Ain't Half Hot Mum* told the tale of a Royal Artillery concert party in Burma at the end of the Second World War and starred Windsor Davies and Melvyn Hayes. *Porridge* with Ronnie Barker was set in the fictional Slade Prison and *Rising Damp* starred Leonard Rossiter as Rigsby, the landlord desperately seeking the attention of Miss Jones, played by Frances de la Tour. It also starred Richard Beckinsale as his student lodger and Don Warrington as the intelligent black lodger.

Wish You Were Here, the travel programme hosted by Judith Chalmers, debuted and elsewhere John Pertwee regenerated into Tom Baker as the fourth *Dr Who*. The last episode of *Monty Python's Flying Circus* was screened this year and the BBC's Ceefax information service began. We were also treated to *Dave Allen at Large*, *Bless This*

Routledge
Taylor & Francis Group

House, *The Benny Hill Show*, and *Sez Les* with Les Dawson and his mother-in-law jokes and dry, moaning sense of humour.

Can you put names to these famous 1970s television catchphrases?

Nice to see you, to see you nice!	Bruce Forsyth
Shut that door!	Larry Grayson
Ooh Betty!	Frank Spencer (Michael Crawford).
You stupid boy!	Captain Mainwaring (Arthur Lowe)
Don't panic!	Corporal Jones (Clive Dunn)
Just like that!	Tommy Cooper
It's the way I tell 'em!	Frank Carson
I'm free!	Mr Humphries (John Inman)
Shoulders back lovely boy!	Windsor Davies
What a wonderful day for …!	Ken Dodd
What do you think of it so far? Rubbish!	Eric Morecambe
Boom Boom!	Basil Brush
Titter ye not!	Frankie Howerd
May your God go with you	Dave Allen

Screen and page

The year's big play was Alan Ayckbourn's *The Norman Conquests*, a trilogy of domestic comedies. In film, Bond returned, with Roger Moore outwitting *The Man with the Golden Gun*, Scaramanga, played by Christopher Lee. Britt Ekland as Miss Goodnight was the love interest. Other big releases were:

Blazing Saddles	Gene Wilder
Chinatown	Jack Nicholson and Faye Dunaway
Towering Inferno	Steve McQueen and Paul Newman
The Great Gatsby	Robert Redford and Mia Farrow

Murder on the Orient Express	Albert Finney and Lauren Bacall
Death Wish	Charles Bronson

The best books this year included John Le Carré's *Tinker, Tailor, Soldier, Spy*, *Carrie* by Stephen King, *Zen and the Art of Motorcycle Maintenance* by Robert M. Pirsig, *The Dispossessed* by Ursula K. Le Guin, and *Switch Bitch* by Roald Dahl.

Sport

Jimmy Connors and Chris Evert won the Wimbledon singles titles. Against all odds, Muhammad Ali regained the world heavyweight title by knocking out George Foreman, seven years his junior, and Britain's John Conteh won the world light heavyweight title.

In football, Manchester United were relegated from the First Division for the first time since 1938. To make matters worse, the relegation was confirmed when they lost to rivals Manchester City 1–0, the goal coming from Denis Law, a former United player!

Liverpool won the FA Cup 3–0 against Newcastle, with Kevin Keegan scoring twice despite Malcolm Macdonald's best efforts! Still with football, World Cup-winning manager Alf Ramsey was sacked after 11 years in charge of the national team. He was succeeded by Don Revie. The football world was then stunned by the announcement that Bill Shankly was stepping down as Liverpool manager after 15 years. He had taken them from the Second Division to First Division and EUFA Cup winners.

Do you remember?

Butlins! Holidays at holiday camps were at a peak and would soon fall victim to cheap overseas package holidays. They were famous for basic chalets, all-inclusive meals and entertainment, and everything being free so that you could have as many rides and goes as possible. Do you remember the redcoats, knobbly knees and bathing beauty contests? There were large outdoor pools and lavish evening variety shows. Many redcoats went on to become famous entertainers, such as Ted Rogers, Des O'Connor and Jimmy Tarbuck. Can you also remember the Butlins enamel badges and those annoying crane-grab slot machines which dropped your prize just before you got it to the hole? What other amusement arcade and slot machines can you recall?

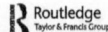

1974 Personal and local events

1975

Major events

January

The 17-year-old heiress Lesley Whittle was kidnapped by Donald Neilson. Her body was found in March in a drain. She had been strangled.

February

Margaret Thatcher defeated Ted Heath to be elected leader of the Conservative Party.

A tube train crash at London's Moorgate station killed 43.

March

Unemployment was in excess of 1 million.

April

Saigon fell to the North Vietnamese and South Vietnam surrendered, effectively ending the Vietnam War.

May

A Japanese woman became the first woman to climb Everest.

After its brakes failed, a runaway coach fell off a bridge at Hebden in Yorkshire, killing the driver and 31 women pensioners on an outing.

June

The Suez Canal reopened after eight years. It was closed during the 1967 Arab–Israeli Six Day War and had to be cleared of mines and sunken ships.

Parliamentary debates were broadcast on the radio for the first time.

July

The USA's *Apollo 18* and the USSR's *Soyuz 19* coupled in space and the crews shared meals in each other's capsules 140 miles above Earth.

August

The 'Birmingham Six' were sentenced to life imprisonment for bombs which killed 21 people in 1974.

A woman was attacked with a hammer in West Yorkshire, the third attack since July.

September

An IRA bomb at the London Hilton killed two people and injured many more.

Czech tennis star Martina Navratilova requested political asylum in the USA.

Having been kidnapped by the Symbionese Liberation Army in February 1974, the heiress Patty Hearst was arrested for armed robbery. She had become a member of the group but claimed she had been brainwashed. She was convicted and jailed until 1979, but in 2001 she was given a pardon by President Bill Clinton.

Dougal Haston and Doug Scott became the first Britons to climb Everest.

The first national museum outside London, the National Railway Museum, opened in York.

November

Pushing a gold-plated button, the Queen started the first flow of North Sea oil near Aberdeen.

British and Icelandic trawlers clashed, marking the beginning of another Cod War.

General Franco of Spain died. He had been the head of state since 1939, when he came to power in the Spanish Civil War. Prince Juan Carlos I was sworn in as King.

December

The Sex Discrimination Act came into force.

Also this year ... inflation was running at nearly 25 per cent and streaking was becoming a familiar sight, with one chap at the Ashes Test Match at Lords jumping over the wicket, spawning many jokes about bails and stumps! The year also brought with it Dutch elm disease, which all but wiped out our native elms. In the USA, Microsoft became a registered trademark with which we were all to become very familiar, and BIC launched the first disposable razor. In electronics, the first digital cameras were being explored, but they were in the early stages of development.

Routledge
Taylor & Francis Group

On the home front

By now more than 25 per cent of the workforce were female, but women were largely in part-time and low-paid employment. Eggs were 40p a dozen, but if you had just over £2,000 you could buy a Vauxhall Cavalier, which was launched this year as a rival to the Ford Cortina.

More and more people were getting telephones, but many still had to walk to the nearest telephone box, invariably in the cold and wet. They usually had a broken window and nearly always someone else was waiting outside, impatient to make their call. A local call was about 2p in the mid-1970s and you were always fearful of running out of coins. For the home the Trimphone arrived in 1975, a slick, modern small phone with a wedge-shaped handpiece; by 1977 it had evolved to have buttons instead of a dial.

Children still played out and their world had not yet shrunk to a bedroom full of games machines and computers. Street games and football were still popular, but for many urban children, building dens was becoming a thing of the past. Many will recall the prospect of enforced cross-country runs at school and by 1975 many local authorities had merged grammar and secondary modern schools into big comprehensives. For sports purposes, many schools were divided into 'houses' which would compete against each other on annual sports days. Uniform policy was somewhat less strict in the comprehensives and it was not unusual to see flared school trousers, tank tops and ties with huge knots in them. For girls, skirt hems were again tending to creep higher.

Music

Ronnie Wood joined the Rolling Stones and Peter Gabriel left Genesis, but heralding a change in musical tastes was the first public performance by the Punk group the Sex Pistols. This year also saw Jamaican Bob Marley spring to fame with his *Natty Dread* album, and Bruce Springsteen with *Born to Run. Bohemian Rhapsody* by Queen went to number one for nine weeks and became the UK's biggest-selling single. Other hits this year included:

Lonely This Christmas	Mud
Make Me Smile (Come Up and See Me)	Steve Harley and Cockney Rebel
Stand By Your Man	Tammy Wynette

 Routledge Taylor & Francis Group

D.I.V.O.R.C.E.	Billy Connolly
Whispering Grass	Don Estelle and Windsor Davies
Sailing	Rod Stewart
Space Oddity	David Bowie
I'm Not in Love	10CC
Down Down	Status Quo
Bye Bye Baby	Bay City Rollers

Television

A popular children's cartoon show was *Scooby Doo* with Shaggy, Fred, Velma and Daphne, who went around solving mysteries in their psychedelic van the 'Mystery Machine'. This was also the year that gave us *Fawlty Towers* with John Cleese as the harassed, erratic and ill-tempered hotel owner Basil Fawlty. His wife Sybil, maid Polly and waiter Manuel ('Que?') made up the cast. Henry Winkler was the Fonz in *Happy Days,* which started this year, as did the drama series *Angels* about nurses, and *Jim'll Fix It* presented by the now-disgraced ex-disc jockey Jimmy Savile. Also debuting was the very popular sitcom *The Good Life* with Tom and Barbara played by Richard Briers and Felicity Kendal, and their posh neighbours Margo and Jerry played by Penelope Keith and Paul Eddington. The police drama *The Sweeney* began with John Thaw as DI Jack Regan and Dennis Waterman as Sergeant George Carter. It was named after the cockney rhyming slang for flying squad, ie, Sweeney Todd!

Screen and page

The film event of the year was undoubtedly filmgoers screaming during screenings of *Jaws*. Other popular films this year included:

Monty Python and the Holy Grail	The *Monty Python* cast
Tommy	Roger Daltrey and Oliver Reed
Picnic at Hanging Rock	Rachel Roberts

Routledge
Taylor & Francis Group

The Man Who Would Be King	Michael Caine and Sean Connery
The Eiger Sanction	Clint Eastwood
The Stepford Wives	Katharine Ross
One Flew Over The Cuckoo's Nest	Jack Nicholson

In literature, *The History Man* by Malcolm Bradbury was published and the first of Colin Dexter's 'Morse' novels, *Last Bus To Woodstock*. Coincidentally, *Morse* was to become a famous role for *Sweeney* actor John Thaw in later years. *The Diaries of a Cabinet Minister* by Richard Crossman was published after a legal battle as the government tried to supress it. Other books were James Clavell's *Shogun*, *The Eagle has Landed* by Jack Higgins and *Salem's Lot* by Stephen King.

Sport

Arthur Ashe became the first black tennis player to win the men's singles at Wimbledon, beating the favourite Jimmy Connors. Austrian Niki Lauda became world motor racing champion and Jack Nicklaus won the US Masters Golf Championship for the fifth time, but at the British Open in Scotland a 25-year-old Tom Watson won.

In football, Brian Clough became manager at Nottingham Forest and his old club Derby County won the League title. West Ham won the FA Cup, beating Fulham 2–0. Riots broke out at the European Cup final as Leeds were beaten 2–0 by Bayern Munich in Paris. UEFA subsequently banned Leeds for a season.

Do you remember?

Seventies sweets such as Bazooka Joe bubble gum, Arrow bars, Old Jamaica chocolate bars, Spangles, Tooty Frooties, Fab and Zoom ice lollies, sweet cigarettes with collectors' cards, Milk Tray chocolate bars, Bar Six, aniseed balls, Munchies and liquorice torpedoes. Can you recall other liquorice sweets, such as pipes and those rolls of liquorice lace with a sweet in the middle?

Routledge
Taylor & Francis Group

1975 Personal and local events

Routledge
Taylor & Francis Group

1976

Major events

January

Hurricane-force winds wreaked havoc across the UK. In three days, over 20 people lost their lives, and many woods were destroyed, cars damaged and roads blocked. Many east coast sea defences were breached, bringing back memories of the terrible events of 1953.

Detective novelist Dame Agatha Christie died aged 85 with some 80 books to her name.

A prostitute was murdered in Leeds as police began to link a series of similar murders.

February

The Winter Olympics at Innsbruck began and John Curry won gold in figure skating.

The Cod War deepened, with Iceland breaking off diplomatic relations with Britain.

March

Prime Minister Harold Wilson resigned after leading the Labour Party for 13 years.

Princess Margaret and Lord Snowden announced they were to separate.

Lord Montgomery, 'Monty' of Alamein, died.

April

James Callaghan became Prime Minister after defeating Roy Jenkins and Michael Foot in the battle for the Labour leadership.

Comedy actor Sid James died of a heart attack on stage in Sunderland.

May

Liberal leader Jeremy Thorpe was forced to resign after allegations of a homosexual relationship with a male model.

Concorde made its first commercial transatlantic flight.

Routledge Taylor & Francis Group

June

Britain and Iceland ended the Cod War.

Three days of rioting occurred in the township of Soweto, South Africa, between blacks and the police after they shot a 13-year-old boy.

A heatwave began which lasted until mid-July, with temperatures reaching over 95 degrees F. Allegedly the driest summer since 1727, it caused a severe drought which triggered water rationing, with hosepipe and car-washing bans.

Palestinian extremists hijacked an Air France plane and forced it to land at Entebbe, Uganda. It was stormed by Israeli commandos on 4 July, freeing all but four of the hostages.

July

David Steel was elected leader of the Liberal Party.

US spacecraft *Viking* landed on Mars and sent back the first pictures of its surface.

A fire destroyed the end of the pier at Southend.

August

Riots spoiled the Notting Hill Carnival.

September

Chinese leader Mao Tse-tung died.

November

One-time peanut farmer Jimmy Carter was elected US President.

Also this year ... the value of fibre in diet was gaining much attention and UK inflation had come down to around 16 per cent. Ironically considering the drought, Rutland Water was opened this year, becoming England's largest reservoir. The National Theatre opened in March, and this was the year that the Tate displayed an 'artistically arranged' pile of bricks, causing a bit of a stir around the question 'What is art?'

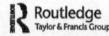
Routledge
Taylor & Francis Group

On the home front

The rear engine Hillman Imp went out of production this year as Ford launched its Fiesta, which was destined to be a very popular family car. It was also a welcome boost to the economy, creating 3,000 jobs at Dagenham. This was the year that the GPO (General Post Office) introduced a mascot called Busby. This yellow cartoon bird pleaded with us to 'Make someone happy with a phone call'. Bernard Cribbins supplied the voice. Remember the GPO used to run the phones as well as the post! This year saw the first branch of Body Shop open in Brighton and the chain soon spread to other major towns, with its ethical perfumes and cosmetics, none of which had been tested on animals. Talking of perfumes, the computer game Pong was at its height. This simulated table tennis: each player had a short line or bat they could move up and down the screen and a small dot (ball) moved from side to side across the screen diagonally. The idea was to move your bat up or down to deflect it back. The ball speeded up as the game progressed until someone missed and then it started slowly speeding up again.

Despite the advent of such modern games, comics and annuals such as the *Beano* and *Dandy* were still well enjoyed. Can you remember these other comics from that era? *Tiger*, *Look-in*, *Valiant*, *Battle*, *Warlord*, *Hotspur*, *Topper*, *Whizzer* and not forgetting *Roy of the Rovers*. Some were educational, such as *Look and Learn*, and the girls had plenty to choose from too, with *Jinty*, *Diana*, *Misty*, *Judy*, *Boyfriend*, *Blue Jeans* and *Jackie*. American DC and Marvel comics were hugely sought-after too, with characters such as Captain America, Spiderman, Hulk, Superman, Batman and Robin, The Fantastic Four and Wonder Woman. There were also the small 'war' comics such as *Commando*. Many comics came with free gifts such as plastic boomerangs, balsa wood gliders, plastic jewellery or jokes such as plastic spiders and fake scars. The American comics had back pages offering tempting mail-order gifts such as X-ray glasses, kryptonite rocks and Sea Monkeys!

Music

British composer Benjamin Britten died this year. Among his best-known works were *Peter Grimes*, *Billy Budd* and *A Young Person's Guide to the Orchestra*. The Eurovision Song Contest was won by Brotherhood of Man with *Save All Your Kisses For Me* and Abba had three number ones with *Dancing Queen*, *Mamma Mia* and *Fernando*.

 Routledge
Taylor & Francis Group

Can you remember who sang these other top pop songs?

If You Leave Me Now	Chicago
Don't Go Breaking My Heart	Elton John and Kiki Dee
December 1963 Oh What a Night	The Four Seasons
Anarchy in the UK	The Sex Pistols
Under the Moon of Love	Showaddywaddy
For Ever and Ever	Demis Roussos
Devil Woman	Cliff Richard
A Little Bit More	Dr Hook
Rhiannon	Fleetwood Mac
You to Me are Everything	The Real Thing
I Love to Love (But My Baby Loves to Dance)	Tina Charles

Can you put names to these significant albums?

Desire	Bob Dylan
A Night at the Opera	Queen
The Song Remains the Same	Led Zeppelin
Songs in the Key of Life	Stevie Wonder
Stupidity	Dr Feelgood

Television

The Muppet Show began, with Kermit the Frog, Miss Piggy, Fozzie Bear, The Great Gonzo and the two old hecklers Waldorf and Statler. Also debuting was *Starsky and Hutch* with David Soul and Paul Michael Glaser and *The Bionic Woman* with Lindsay Wagner. The drama series *When the Boat Comes In*, starring James Bolam, was a gritty North East drama centred around a First World War veteran returning to his home. Also beginning was *Multi-Coloured Swap Shop* with Noel Edmonds, Keith

Routledge
Taylor & Francis Group

Chegwin, Maggie Philbin and John Craven. It was rivalled by *Tiswas* with Chris Tarrant, Lenny Henry and Sally James. *Open All Hours* with Ronnie Barker as Arkwright the grocer and David Jason his assistant Granville was also a newcomer. The other well-loved comedy to emerge this year was *George and Mildred* starring Yootha Joyce and Brian Murphy. Its plot was essentially around the fraught relationship of the bickering couple who move to a 'posh' estate and a neighbour who thinks they lower the tone of the area. The Punk band The Sex Pistols achieved notoriety by swearing on television on *The Bill Grundy Show*, though the presenter had goaded them into doing so. This was also the year in which Rod Hull's Emu attacked Michael Parkinson on his chat show.

Screen and page

Books published this year included *Roots* by Alex Haley, *Wilt* by Tom Sharpe, *The Selfish Gene* by Richard Dawkins, *Not a Penny More, Not a Penny Less* by Jeffrey Archer and Agatha Christie's final novel, the last in the Miss Marple series, *Sleeping Murder.*

This year's best films included:

Taxi Driver	Robert De Niro
A Star is Born	Barbra Streisand and Kris Kristofferson
Rocky	Sylvester Stallone
The Omen	Gregory Peck
Logan's Run	Michael York and Jenny Agutter
All The President's Men	Robert Redford and Dustin Hoffman
The Outlaw Josey Wales	Clint Eastwood
The Man Who Fell To Earth	David Bowie
Bugsy Malone	Jodie Foster

… and a remake of *King Kong* with Jessica Lange.

Routledge
Taylor & Francis Group

Sport

Which British driver became the world Formula One champion?
James Hunt

Which figure skater carried off the British, European, World and Olympic titles?
John Curry

Which Swede became the youngest Wimbledon men's singles champion for 45 years?
He beat Ilie Nastase and went on to win Wimbledon for the next four years.
Bjorn Borg (aged 20)

At the Olympic Games in Montreal, which 14-year-old competing on the asymmetrical bars got the first perfect 10 ever awarded in gymnastics and went on to get another six perfect 10s, gaining her three golds, a silver and a bronze?   *Nadia Comaneci*

Meanwhile, Great Britain and Northern Ireland won three golds including the 200m breaststroke won by …?   *David Wilkie*

Second Division Southampton beat Manchester United 1–0 in the FA Cup final. Who was United's manager at the time?   *Tommy Docherty*

Which team won the UEFA Cup for the second time, beating Belgians FC Brugge KV?
Liverpool

Who won the World Snooker Championship, beating Alex 'Hurricane' Higgins 27–16?
Ray Reardon

Which 22-year-old Austrian prodigy won an Olympic gold medal in downhill skiing?
He had won the world downhill title in 1975 and went on to win it in 1976, 1977, 1978 and 1983.   *Franz Klammer*

Do you remember?

These 1970s toys: Etch-a-Sketch, Stylophone, Spirograph, Superballs, Sillystring, Crossfire, Buckaroo, Dymotape label printers and Kerplunk. Skateboarding was also just becoming very popular, as were Hotwheels, with long stretches of plastic track where you could make your car jump long gaps and do stunts and loop the loops! However, old favourites were still popular and Airfix model kits were still on most boys' Christmas lists as the range was expanded to include spacecraft and larger-scale models. How many of us remember brothers or friends whose bedroom ceilings had Airfix planes hanging from them, dive bombing each other?

1976 Personal and local events

Routledge
Taylor & Francis Group

1977

Major events

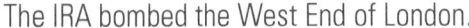

January
The US restored the death penalty and executed Gary Gilmore, a double murderer, by firing squad.

The IRA bombed the West End of London.

The Pompidou Centre in Paris opened, rivalling the Eiffel Tower as an architectural innovation. Brightly coloured and transparent tubes carried the services and escalators around the outside of the building.

February
Another woman was murdered in Leeds and the police linked it to three other murders and three attempted ones.

March
The Queen's Jubilee tour reached Australia and the centenary Test Match between England and Australia began in Melbourne. Australia won both matches.

Large numbers of British Leyland workers went on strike and the government threatened to withdraw state aid to the company. The government subsequently lost the confidence of the House of Commons and Prime Minister Callaghan was forced to make a pact with Liberal leader David Steel.

Two jumbo jets collided on the runway in Tenerife, killing 582.

April
A woman was murdered in Bradford. She was believed to be another victim of the serial killer the press were now calling the Yorkshire Ripper.

June
A public holiday for the Queen's Silver Jubilee saw many people holding street parties.

Leonid Brezhnev was named USSR President and Communist Party leader. He took over from Nikita Khrushchev.

Police clashed with trade union pickets and demonstrators outside Grunwick film laboratories in London. Flying pickets from the Yorkshire coalfields attended the demonstration, along with their leader Arthur Scargill and many other union delegations. The dispute about trade union recognition lasted two years in total.

Another 'Ripper' victim was found in Leeds.

August
'The King is Dead!' The legendary singer Elvis Presley was found dead aged 42. Dubbed 'The King of Rock and Roll', his death caused a huge outpouring of grief by fans. By his last year he was a caricature of his former Rock and Roll image, only 42 but grossly overweight and suffering a multitude of other ailments allegedly brought on by drug abuse. Many gathered outside Graceland, his mansion in Tennessee, to view his open casket. Conspiracy theorists suggested he faked his own death so that he could retire in peace, sparking the occasional tabloid headline 'Elvis is alive'! If you have a copy of the newspaper from the day proclaiming 'Elvis is dead', you might be richer than you think!

September
Black South African Leader Steve Biko (30) was found dead with brain injuries during police detention in Port Elizabeth, South Africa, sparking anti-police demonstrations and unrest.

Glam Rock pop star Marc Bolan was killed in a car crash at the age of 29.

Freddie Laker's cheap airline Skytrain was launched, undercutting the competition. He was knighted a year later.

October
Police launched an appeal for help in finding the Yorkshire Ripper.

November
Firefighters went on strike for the first time, looking for a 30 per cent wage rise. The troops were quickly brought in with their 'Green Goddesses'.

December
Disaster struck. The England football team did not qualify for the World Cup for the second time in succession.

A London Underground extension to Heathrow was opened.

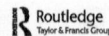

Also this year …. there was civil war in Angola and much unrest in Rhodesia, Uganda and Ethiopia. The Queen toured the Commonwealth in her Silver Jubilee year, being welcomed by large crowds. Merchandising went mad and you could buy Jubilee versions of nearly everything from biscuits to margarine! There was even a fizzy drink called Jubilade! Those who felt it was all a bit too much could buy a 'Stuff the Jubilee' badge.

On the home front

As Punk was taking hold, one of the fashion travesties of the 1970s was at its height. Feathered haircuts had been popular since the early 1970s, but became even more so when Farrah Fawcett-Majors shot to fame sporting one in *Charlie's Angels*. A shorter version for men, not a million miles away from the 'mullet', was popularised by the Bay City Rollers.

Bowing to the pressure from the anti-smoking lobby, tobacco companies introduced NSM or New Smoking Material. This was a lower nicotine cigarette, but it just didn't catch on. What did catch on were the Pot Noodles and snack pots which came on the scene, with many people finding them convenient as an alternative to a packed lunch.

Over a million skateboards were sold in the UK this year. A way of 'surfing' on land, these American toys were a very familiar sight in the streets. In the motoring world, foreign cars were now outselling British ones, with makes such as Renault and Volkswagen and Japanese cars such as Datsuns. Shopping was changing too, with the popularisation of home shopping from catalogues such as Littlewoods and Freemans. Fashion, kitchenware, furniture, electrical goods, and so on all could be bought conveniently from the comfort of your armchair. They were popular because you could spread the cost by paying by instalments.

Music

As well as Marc Bolan, the music industry lost three other giants this year, Elvis on 16 August, opera diva Maria Callas on 17 September and crooner and star, with Bob Hope, of the 'Road to' movies, Bing Crosby, on 14 October. Crosby had recorded *Peace on Earth/Little Drummer Boy* with David Bowie just five weeks earlier. It was to be a hit in 1982 when it was rediscovered. Popular hits this year included:

Don't Cry For Me Argentina	Julie Covington
I Love To Boogie	T. Rex
I Don't Want to Talk About it/ The First Cut is the Deepest	Rod Stewart
I Feel Love	Donna Summer
Chanson d'Amour	Manhattan Transfer
We are the Champions	Queen
When I Need You	Leo Sayer
Rockin' All Over the World	Status Quo
Way Down	Elvis Presley
Yes Sir, I Can Boogie	Baccara
Mull of Kintyre	Wings
Knowing Me, Knowing You	Abba
Black is Black	La Belle Epoque

Many of the albums of the 1970s were of the 'greatest hits' variety, but the album *Never Mind the Bollocks, Here's the Sex Pistols* confirmed that the Punk era had arrived, with its attendant fashions and hairstyles. Other albums this year included one of the best-selling albums of all time, *Rumours* by Fleetwood Mac. Others were:

Arrival	Abba
Hotel California	The Eagles
Exodus	Bob Marley and the Wailers
Animals	Pink Floyd
Songs in the Key of Life	Stevie Wonder
Rattus Norvegicus	The Stranglers

Routledge Taylor & Francis Group

Television

This year saw the start of the comedy series *Citizen Smith* with Robert 'power to the people' Lindsay. There were also two new action dramas, *Charlie's Angels* played by Farrah Fawcett-Majors, Kate Jackson and Jaclyn Smith and *The Professionals* with the characters Bodie and Doyle. Robert Powell played Jesus in the drama series *Jesus of Nazareth* and Des O'Connor began a successful run with his variety show *Des O'Connor Tonight*. The first *It'll Be Alright on the Night*, presented by Denis Norden, was aired this year.

Coronation Street took part in the Jubilee celebrations with the street entering a float in the Weatherfield Jubilee parade. With the theme of 'Britain Through the Ages', Rovers Return landlady Annie Walker was Queen Elizabeth I, Bet Lynch the barmaid was Britannia and Ena Sharples was Queen Victoria, while Eddie Yeats was a caveman. Stan Ogden was to drive the float but left the lights on all night, draining the battery, so everyone missed the parade.

Screen and page

Can you remember who starred in this year's must-see films?

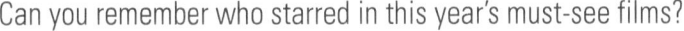

Close Encounters of the Third Kind	Richard Dreyfuss
Saturday Night Fever	John Travolta
Star Wars	Mark Hamill, Carrie Fisher and Harrison Ford
Annie Hall	Woody Allen and Diane Keaton
The Spy Who Loved Me	Roger Moore and Barbara Bach
Smokey and the Bandit	Burt Reynolds and Sally Field
A Bridge Too Far	Sean Connery and Michael Caine
The Deep	Jaqueline Bisset
Equus	Richard Burton
The Rescuers	A cartoon about mice searching for a little girl.

 Routledge Taylor & Francis Group

This year also saw the premiere of Mike Leigh's play *Abigail's Party*. This play was a satire on the social mores of the aspiring middle class of the decade. It starred the flirty Alison Steadman as Demis Roussos-loving Beverly. With her aspiring estate agent husband Lawrence she holds a party for new neighbours Tony and his drippy wife Angela. Another neighbour, Susan, is invited, who is worried about her daughter Abigail, at home having a party.

In literature, books published included Patrick Leigh Fermor's *A Time of Gifts*, Bruce Chatwin's *In Patagonia*, John Fowles' *Daniel Martin*, J. R. R. Tolkien's *The Silmarillion*, Colleen McCullough's *The Thorn Birds* and Edith Holden's *The Country Diary of an Edwardian Lady*.

Sport

Geoff Boycott returned to Test cricket with a century against the Australians at Trent Bridge and then again for his 100th century at his home ground of Headingly. The cricket authorities in Australia and England were upset this year as Kerry Packer set up a rival World Test Match series. Elsewhere, Red Rum won the Grand National for the third time and, as the Queen celebrated her Jubilee, she was able to watch Virginia Wade take the Wimbledon women's title at her 13th attempt. The Embassy World Snooker Championship moved to its spiritual home at the Crucible Theatre in Sheffield, where it was televised for the first time. Tobacco company sponsorship was not yet an issue!

In football, Liverpool won the League for the tenth time and Tommy Docherty was sacked as Manchester United manager for having an affair with the wife of the club's physiotherapist. He was replaced by Dave Sexton. Manchester United went on to beat Liverpool 2–1 to win the FA Cup. Liverpool's sorrows did not last long, as four days later they won the European Cup, beating Borussia Monchengladbach 3–1 in Rome. Later in September they were to be temporarily kicked out of the European Cup Winners' Cup after fans rioted in the first round. Kenny Dalglish became Britain's most expensive footballer when he was transferred to Liverpool from Celtic for £440,000, and Don Revie resigned as England manager to take up a lucrative offer to manage the United Arab Emirates. He was succeeded by Ron Greenwood despite many wanting Brian Clough to get the job.

Routledge
Taylor & Francis Group

Do you remember?

Punk! With the success and notoriety of the Sex Pistols and other Punk bands, Punk culture and fashion were becoming a familiar sight. Ripped T-shirts and safety pins holding clothes together went alongside brightly coloured Mohican haircuts and bin liners for shirts! Spiky hair, studs in jackets and safety pins through noses as well as spitting at each other while dancing the 'pogo' were all part of the movement. Punks saw themselves as outside and against mainstream society and their music was typically angry and basic. Their rebellious attitudes and anti-fashion clothes represented a statement against the prevailing norms of society. However, in the grand scheme of things the Punk 'revolution' was a sign of normality … haven't teenagers always rebelled? Remember the Teddy Boys and Mods and Rockers! Eventually Punk was commercialised and many of the bands went on to fame and glory … or sold out!

1977 Personal and local events

Routledge
Taylor & Francis Group

1978

Major events

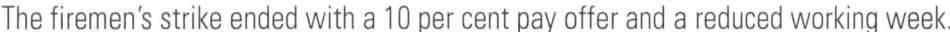

January

A storm wrecked Skegness, Hunstanton, Herne Bay and Margate piers.

The firemen's strike ended with a 10 per cent pay offer and a reduced working week.

Margaret Thatcher fanned the flames of prejudice by suggesting that many in the country feared being 'swamped' by people with a different culture. However, such sentiments brought about a change in Tory fortunes as they moved ahead of Labour in the polls.

Another Yorkshire Ripper victim was found.

March

Supertanker *Amoco Cadiz* ran aground off Brittany, losing 220,000 tonnes of crude oil and fouling more than 100 miles of French coastline.

The Conservatives recruited advertising agency Saatchi and Saatchi to revamp their image.

May

May Day became a Bank Holiday for the first time.

The 10th Ripper victim was found in Manchester.

July

Louise Brown, the world's first test-tube baby, was born at Oldham General Hospital.

August

Pope Paul VI died, to be replaced by John Paul I. On 28 September he suddenly died too, and was replaced by Cardinal Karol Wojtyla as John Paul II, the first non-Italian Pope since 1523.

Routledge
Taylor & Francis Group

September

The Lib–Lab pact was ended by Prime Minister James Callaghan, who refused to call an autumn election despite now heading a minority government, as the polls put Labour ahead again.

Bulgarian defector Georgi Markov was murdered in London, by being stabbed in the thigh with an umbrella which embedded a poisoned pellet in his leg.

Strikes closed 26 Ford car plants across Britain.

October

Liverpool Cathedral was completed. Its foundation stone had been laid in 1934.

November

A bakers' strike led to panic buying and rationing.

Followers of the Reverend Jim Jones committed mass suicide in Guyana, when 909 people, including 303 children, drank cyanide.

A Birmingham night club was forced by the Commission for Racial Equality to end its entry policy of barring black and Chinese people.

Viv Anderson became the first black England international footballer.

Industrial action closed *The Times* newspaper, which did not reappear until November 1979. This strike was one of many as the Labour government tried to control inflation by keeping pay rises down. The Trades Union Congress (TUC) opposed these measures and, in what was to be a very cold winter, supported a series of strikes including those by refuse collectors, lorry and tanker drivers, and railway and car workers. As rubbish piled up in the streets and petrol supplies became scarce, the government's popularity dwindled. The strikes lasted until February 1979 and largely paved the way for the following year's Conservative election victory. By the end of the year inflation was down to just over 8 per cent but unemployment was at a post-war high of 1.5 million.

Also this year … Sweden was the first country to ban the use of aerosols because of their impact upon the environment. Compact discs were first demonstrated; concrete cows were erected in Milton Keynes as part of an art project; and a 'winter of discontent' loomed large.

Routledge
Taylor & Francis Group

On the home front

By 1978 most of us had colour televisions, and VHS (video home system) recorders went on sale for the first time this year. These machines took large black book-sized cassettes and quickly became popular. As the ownership of recorders grew, so did the number of video hire shops, and it soon became a cheap 'night out' to stay in with a video instead!

It has been suggested that in 1978 the world's quality of life peaked. In the UK life was good for many, but for others it was not so good, with unemployment at a post-war high of 1.5 million. But for those in employment there had never been more technical gadgetry to buy for the home, and culturally there was a feelgood factor with the disco era ('Grease is the word!') and flamboyant fashions. The prevailing politics lacked this optimism, though. It was the year which gave us 'Rock Against Racism'. The National Front was becoming prominent and there were often clashes with the Anti-Nazi League on marches. Prominent anti-Nazi performers were Tom Robinson, Elvis Costello and The Clash and many cities held anti-Nazi concerts. This was the year of the 'sus' laws, when many blacks were arrested 'on suspicion of the intent to commit an offence', so it was not surprising that there were clashes between black youths and the police. On a more positive note, many bands with mixed race line-ups such as The Specials were emerging, helping to combat the racism.

Back at school and too young to be aware of the politics, the craze among the swots was for pocket calculators. One calculator trick was to make up words from the letters and symbols on the display screen. If you typed in 8075 and turned it upside down you had SLOB. Needless to say, there were many worse such words that 'clever' pupils could come up with!

Music

James Galway's flute music was popular and his *Annie's Song* was a huge hit. However, *Mull of Kintyre* by Wings became the biggest-selling single in UK history. Kate Bush arrived on the scene, and the year's hits included:

Take a Chance on Me	Abba
Wuthering Heights	Kate Bush

Rivers of Babylon	Boney M
You're the One That I Want	Olivia Newton John and John Travolta
Summer Nights	Olivia Newton John and John Travolta
Three Times a Lady	The Commodores
Dreadlock Holiday	10CC
Do Ya Think I'm Sexy?	Rod Stewart
Baker Street	Gerry Rafferty
YMCA	Village People
Stayin' Alive	Bee Gees
Mister Blue Sky	Electric Light Orchestra
Matchstick Men and Matchstick Cats and Dogs	Brian and Michael

Of the albums this year, the soundtrack to *Saturday Night Fever* sold the most, but *Bat Out of Hell* by Meatloaf sold around 48 million copies worldwide and became a Rock classic.

Television

The soap opera *Crossroads* was at the height of its popularity and the original series of *Top Gear* aired on BBC2. It had begun life as a regional programme the previous year.

Beginning this year was the television version of James Herriot's Yorkshire vet tales *All Creatures Great and Small*. It starred Christopher Timothy as James, Robert Hardy as his boss Siegfried and Peter Davidson as his younger brother Tristan. Another notable debut came in the form of the very popular children's programme *Grange Hill*. Culturally, we saw the start of *The South Bank Show* presented by Melvyn Bragg. Less culturally, we had the quiz show *3-2-1* with Ted Rogers and Dusty Bin, the show's booby prize!

Anna Ford became ITN's first female newsreader and talent shows were very popular. We had Hughie 'and I mean that most sincerely folks' Green's *Opportunity Knocks* with

Routledge
Taylor & Francis Group

its 'clapometer' measuring audience appreciation, and *New Faces*, which had a panel judging the acts. Many household names got their breaks via these programmes, for instance Lenny Henry, Victoria Wood, Paul Daniels, Les Dawson and Lena Zavaroni.

On radio, 8 March saw the first episode of *The Hitchhiker's Guide to the Galaxy*, which later became a bestselling book.

Screen and page

On stage we had Tim Rice and Andrew Lloyd Webber's musical *Evita*, about Eva Peron, and in the cinema the year's favourite releases included:

Superman	Christopher Reeve
The Deer Hunter	Robert De Niro and Christopher Walken
Grease	Olivia Newton John and John Travolta
Halloween	Donald Pleasance and Jamie Lee Curtis
Midnight Express	Brad Davis
Watership Down	Bigwig, Hazel and Fiver!
Every Which Way But Loose	Clint Eastwood
The Wild Geese	Richard Harris, Richard Burton and Roger Moore
The Thirty Nine Steps	Robert Powell

and … *Attack of the Killer Tomatoes*!

In books, we had Graham Greene's *The Human Factor*, Frederick Forsyth's *The Day of the Jackal*, M. Scott Peck's *The Road Less Travelled*, Raymond Briggs' *The Snowman* and M. M. Kaye's *The Far Pavilions*.

Sport

Can you solve these 1978 sporting conundrums?

Who, at the age of 22, became the first man since Fred Perry to win the Wimbledon men's singles title three times in a row?   *Bjorn Borg*

Six years after taking Derby County to the League title, who took their Midlands rivals there as Nottingham Forest won the League?   *Brian Clough*

Who was the only other manager to have done this in the inter-war years, with Huddersfield and Arsenal?   *Herbert Chapman*

Who won the FA Cup for the first time, beating Arsenal 1–0?   *Ipswich Town*

Who retained the European Cup, beating Brugge KV at Wembley?   *Liverpool*

Who won the World Cup in Argentina, beating the Netherlands 3–1?   *Argentina*

In cricket, who became the first man in Test history to hit a century and take eight wickets in one innings?   *Ian Botham*

Who became the first woman to sail around the world single-handed?   *Naomi James*

Who lost his world heavyweight title to Leon Spinks, then beat him in a rematch to become the first boxer to win the title three times?   *Muhammad Ali*

Do you remember?

LPs were around £2.49p and singles about 79p! There were also cheaper LPs from 'Music for Pleasure' and a series of *Top of the Pops* LPs on the Hallmark label. They had cover versions of recent hits and always had a cover with a scantily-clad girl on. This was also the era of disco, which conjures up images of 1970s' man strutting his stuff on the dance floor in tight trousers, with shirt open to the navel and a medallion hanging on his manly chest! Ask group members to recall their own worst dance embarrassments!

Routledge
Taylor & Francis Group

1978 Personal and local events

Routledge
Taylor & Francis Group

1979

Major events

January

Vietnam invaded Cambodia, ending the tyrannical rule of Pol Pot and the Khmer Rouge.

The 'winter of discontent' continued, with lorry drivers' strikes, schools forced to close because of lack of heating oil, and industrial unrest. As Prime Minister Callaghan returned from overseas and played down the situation, the *Sun* newspaper reported his comments with the headline 'Crisis? What crisis?'

After months of demonstrations the ruling Shah was forced to leave Iran and was replaced by the religious leader Ayatollah Khomeini. People later voted strongly for an Islamic Republic.

February

Sex Pistols guitarist Sid Vicious died at 21 from a heroin overdose.

March

Devolution referendums were held in Wales and Scotland. Scotland voted 'for' but not enough people voted to make it count, and Wales vote 'against'.

Conservative Northern Ireland spokesman Airey Neave was killed by an IRA car bomb as he left the House of Commons underground car park.

April

Another Ripper victim was found in Halifax.

Ugandan self-styled President Idi Amin was finally deposed after eight years in power, ending his regime of terror.

The first 'one man, one vote' elections took place in Rhodesia, electing the first black Prime Minister, Bishop Abel Muzorewa.

Anti-Nazi League protester Blair Peach was killed by a police truncheon blow.

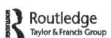

May

Margaret Thatcher was elected as the first female British Prime Minister when the Conservatives won the general election. Liberal Jeremy Thorpe lost his seat. By the end of May the Conservatives had outlined plans to sell off nationalised industries.

The government agreed to take in fleeing Vietnamese boat people picked up in the South China Sea.

June

The first elections took place for Members of the European Parliament (MEPs).

US actor John Wayne died.

July

In Iran, after having returned from a 16-year exile on 1 February, Ayatollah Khomeini banned the broadcasting of music.

August

Disgraced MP John Stonehouse was released from prison.

Earl Mountbatten of Burma, the Queen's cousin, was murdered by the IRA when they blew up his boat. Eighteen British soldiers were killed in Northern Ireland the same day.

September

The 20th Yorkshire Ripper victim was found in Bradford.

Lord Mountbatten's funeral took place at Westminster Abbey.

Much-loved wartime singer Gracie Fields died. Her most famous song was *Sally*.

Pope John Paul II visited Ireland.

November

Ayatollah Khomeini supporters occupied the US Embassy in Tehran, holding 52 people hostage inside.

The Times newspaper reappeared after nearly a year following an industrial dispute.

December

Stunt rider Eddie Kidd, aged 20, leapt an 80-foot gap at 90 mph on a motorcycle.

Routledge
Taylor & Francis Group

Also this year … the Nobel Peace Prize was won by Mother Teresa for work in the slums of Calcutta; the first Wetherspoons pub opened in London; and the Sony Walkman was launched in Japan, although it was a few years before it became the popular must-have gadget. With inflation running at 13.4 per cent, the Conservative government pushed through billions of pounds in public spending cuts. The year was also notable for achieving the highest number of days lost through strike action since 1926.

On the home front

Skinhead culture was just coming back in fashion. Emerging from the Mod fashions of the 1950s and 1960s, it was to become associated with violence. Dr Marten boots and braces were worn over Ben Sherman shirts and jeans were worn short with turn-ups. Many working class youths suffering high unemployment and poverty turned to fascist movements such as the National Front and the football terraces to vent their anger.

For those in the money, milk had risen to 15p a pint and in November Vauxhall introduced the Astra range of family cars, replacing the old Vauxhall Viva. The great shopping boom was further fuelled on 25 September when Margaret Thatcher opened the new shopping centre in Milton Keynes. It was the largest in the UK.

Food tastes were also changing and we were treated to such modern delights as Arctic Roll. Breville sandwich toasters were also popular now. They were often used furiously for a few weeks and then ignored because no one bothered to clean them! By the end of the 1970s much more frozen food could be had and fast food was becoming ever more popular, with Wimpy Bars proliferating in this pre-McDonald's era. A cheeseburger would set you back about 25p!

Music

This year's hit singles included:

Hit Me With Your Rhythm Stick	Ian Dury and the Blockheads
Bright Eyes	Art Garfunkel
I Don't Like Mondays	The Boomtown Rats
Message in a Bottle	The Police

Walking on the Moon	The Police
Video Killed the Radio Star	Buggles
Another Brick in the Wall	Pink Floyd
We Don't Talk Anymore	Cliff Richard
I Will Survive	Gloria Gaynor
Cars	Gary Numan
Tragedy	The Bee Gees
Crazy Little Thing Called Love	Queen
Heart of Glass	Blondie
Cool for Cats	Squeeze
When You're in Love with a Beautiful Woman	Dr Hook
Eton Rifles	The Jam

Can you also put names to these best-selling albums?

Parallel Lines	Blondie
Voulez-Vous	Abba
Tusk	Fleetwood Mac
The Great Rock and Roll Swindle	The Sex Pistols

Television

The Yorkshire farming community soap opera *Emmerdale Farm* began this year, as did *Tales of the Unexpected*, based on Roald Dahl's adult short stories. Robin Day presented the first *Question Time* and other debuts included *Blankety Blank*, *Antiques Roadshow*, *Not the Nine O'Clock News*, *Terry and June*, *Worzel Gummidge*, and the very popular *To The Manor Born* with Penelope Keith and Peter Bowles. Can you also remember *Mork and Mindy* with Robin Williams as Mork from Ork, whose catchphrase was 'nanu nanu'?

Routledge
Taylor & Francis Group

David Attenborough's *Life on Earth* was a hugely successful wildlife series and famously saw him being groomed by a family of gorillas. The wacky gameshow *It's a Knockout* was at the height of its popularity with its weird challenges. Teams representing towns competed against each other in silly games, usually in fancy dress and usually involving water. Each team could play their 'Joker' and get double points if they won that game. Its international version, *Jeux Sans Frontières*, was also a success.

Can you recall the *Morecambe and Wise Christmas Show*? This was something of a national institution in the 1970s. Every Christmas Day saw a Morecambe and Wise special. They were at the height of their popularity and the show always ended with a big theatrical production 'what Ernie wrote'! These invariably took the mickey out of their special guests. Notable Christmas specials involved Penelope Keith being unceremoniously manhandled and putting her feet through the stage, Eric as a policeman getting soaked as Ernie danced to *Singing in the Rain*, Eric calling the conductor André Previn Mr Preview and, when challenged that he was playing Grieg's piano concerto wrongly, said, 'I'm playing all the right notes but not necessarily in the right order'! The pair also once had BBC newsreaders dancing and singing *There Ain't Nothing Like a Dame* and doing somersaults, but perhaps their most famous sketch was the one in which newsreader Angela Rippon emerged from behind her desk in a leg-revealing gown and began a high-kicking song and dance routine.

Screen and page

This year's best sellers included *Moortown* by the poet Ted Hughes, *The Hitchhiker's Guide to the Galaxy* by Douglas Adams, *A Bend in the River* by V. S. Naipaul, *Sophie's Choice* by William Styron, *Tales of the Unexpected* by Roald Dahl and *A Woman of Substance* by Barbara Taylor Bradford.

Can you remember who starred in this year's popular film releases?

Alien	Sigourney Weaver
Apocalypse Now	Marlon Brando and Martin Sheen
Mad Max	Mel Gibson
Manhattan	Woody Allen and Diane Keaton
The Life of Brian	The Monty Python cast

10	Dudley Moore and Bo Derrick
Kramer vs Kramer	Meryl Streep and Dustin Hoffman
Moonraker	Roger Moore
Yanks	Richard Gere
Being There	Peter Sellers and Shirley MacLaine

As a tribute to John Wayne, who died this year, how many John Wayne films can you name? They include *Stagecoach*, *Reap the Wild Wind*, *Red River*, *Sands of Iwo Jima*, *The Quiet Man* and *True Grit*.

Sport

Sebastian Coe became the first man to hold all 800 metres, 1500 metres and mile world records. In July he broke the world mile record, taking it down to 3 minutes 48.95 seconds. In cricket, Australian Jeff Thomson was recorded as the fastest Test bowler in the world. In football, manager Brian Clough signed Trevor Francis for Nottingham Forest making him Britain's first £1 million footballer. He scored the only goal in Nottingham Forest's European Cup Final against Malmo, thus making his transfer fee worthwhile. This was quite an achievement for 'Forest', who were only two seasons out of the Second Division. In the FA Cup, Arsenal beat Manchester United 3–2.

Tragically, a storm hit the Fastnet yachting race, the last event in the Admiral's Cup. Five yachts sank and 15 lives were lost in the tempestuous seas and gale force winds.

Do you remember?

See if you can remember these classic 1970s television adverts and their slogans!

And all because the lady loves … *Milk Tray*

I won't be there when you cross the road so always use the … *Green Cross Code*

She flies like a bird in the sky *Nimble*

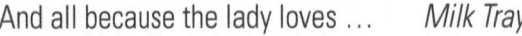

Lipsmackinthirstquenchinacetastinmotivatinggoodbuzzincooltalkinhighwalkinfastlivinever givincoolfizzin *Pepsi*

Routledge
Taylor & Francis Group

For mash get … *Smash*

I'd like to teach the world to sing in perfect harmony *Coca Cola*

Made in Scotland from girders *Irn Bru*

Naughty but nice *Fresh cream cakes*

Is she or isn't she? *Harmony hairspray*

Full of Eastern promise *Fry's Turkish Delight*

A drink's too wet without one *Rich Tea biscuits*

Building houses to make homes in *Barratt*

Only the crumbliest, flakiest chocolate tastes like chocolate never tasted before *Cadbury's Flake*

Can you also recall those PG Tips adverts with the chimpanzees? They started in the 1950s and were dropped in the mid 1970s because of animal rights complaints, but as sales declined they were quickly resuscitated. 'Dad, do you know the piano's on my foot?', 'You hum it son, I'll play it', 'Avez-vous un cuppa?'

1979 Personal and local events

1980

Major events

January
Steelworkers went on strike for the first time since 1926 in a bid to get a 20 per cent rise.

February
British Steel announced 11,000 jobs were to go in Wales.

March
Robert Mugabe was elected Prime Minister of Zimbabwe, which became independent on 18 April.

Pirate radio station Radio Caroline had to cease transmission when the ship where it was based sank!

The government wanted to stop athletes competing at the Olympic Games in Moscow but the British Olympic Association defied them.

Robert Runcie was enthroned as Archbishop of Canterbury.

A fairly typical Budget saw the government both give and take by raising tax allowances but also raising the duty on petrol, tobacco and alcohol.

April
The steelworkers' strike was called off.

Spain reopened its border with UK territory Gibraltar.

Philosopher Jean-Paul Sartre died aged 74.

President Carter launched a raid to release the US Embassy hostages being held in Iran since November 1979. It went disastrously wrong.

Armed terrorists seized the Iranian Embassy in London, taking 26 hostages.

May

British Aerospace was privatised.

The SAS stormed the Iranian Embassy in London, rescuing the hostages and killing five terrorists. They used stun grenades and dramatically abseiled down the walls and swung in through the windows.

June

The pre-decimal sixpence was withdrawn from circulation. The 'tanner' was no longer!

July

Alexandra Palace was gutted by fire.

The film star and 'Goon' Peter Sellers died aged 54.

August

Polish shipyard workers under the leadership of Lech Walesa went on strike, demanding free trade unions and an end to press censorship. Later in the month they were allowed to form their union and call it 'Solidarity'.

September

CND held a rally at Greenham Common in protest at the siting of US nuclear missiles there.

October

Council house tenants got the right to buy their homes.

Margaret Thatcher made her famous 'The lady's not for turning' speech in reference to criticisms from her own party's MPs that her economic policy was fuelling the recession. Union leaders were also critical and warned of civil unrest.

James Callaghan resigned as leader of the Labour Party.

The Queen became the first British monarch to make a state visit to the Vatican.

November

Ronald Reagan was elected US President.

Michael Foot was elected leader of the Labour Party.

A 20-year-old female university student was murdered in Leeds, another suspected 'Ripper' victim.

December
John Lennon was shot dead outside his apartment in New York.

Also this year … the population was now around 56 million. The new decade began with a recession due to unemployment at a post-war high of over 1 million and inflation at nearly 22 per cent. We lost the tanner but we got 'post it' notes!

On the home front

The Austin Metro was launched this year. The small hatchback was similar to the Mini but it had slightly more space inside. It was designed to be an economy car and was popular enough to outsell Ford's Fiesta, though it was a little prone to rust. It retailed at over £6,000, which was just about the average annual salary. The average weekly wage was around £127.70 for men but just £75.50 for women. Britain was in a deep recession in mid-1980. Petrol was 28p a litre, a first class stamp 12p and beer around 35p a pint, 2p more than a loaf of bread but cheap by today's standards. On the fashion front, Kickers shoes were 'in' and jeans were still popular, but flares had long gone in favour of stonewashed straight-leg jeans. Loose shirts for men were on their way in as we headed towards the 'New Romantic' age!

The must-have toy was the Rubik's Cube. This was a three-dimensional puzzle in the form of a cube with nine coloured squares on each face. The faces could be turned independently and so got very mixed up; the hard bit was getting them back so that each face only had one colour. The other soon-to-be craze was for the arcade game Pac-Man. Basically, you guided Pac-Man through a maze, eating Pac-dots as you went. Sounds easy, but there were enemies in the maze who ate you! If you ate as many dots as you could and didn't lose any lives you could move up to the next level. It became a 1980s phenomenon and addiction, with huge merchandising spin-offs.

Music

Ska and Two Tone music was in vogue, with The Specials, Madness and UB40 having hits this year. The bands featured a mixture of black and white musicians. Kate Bush became the first British female to have a number one album, *Never for Ever*, and Cliff Richard was given an MBE.

This year's best-selling singles included:

Kings of the Wild Frontier	Adam and the Ants
Another Brick in the Wall	Pink Floyd
Brass in Pocket	The Pretenders
Going Underground	The Jam
Geno	Dexy's Midnight Runners
Ashes to Ashes	David Bowie
The Tide is High	Blondie
Super Trouper	Abba
Working My Way Back to You	Detroit Spinners
Baggy Trousers	Madness
To Cut a Long Story Short	Spandau Ballet
Don't Stand So Close to Me	The Police

Television

This year's debuts included *Hi De Hi*, set in the fictional Maplins holiday camp. It starred Sue Pollard as Peggy the chalet maid, Ruth Madoc as Gladys Pugh the sports organiser, Simon Cadell as the entertainment manager and Paul Shane as Ted Bovis, the camp host and yellow coat. The other new comedy this year was *Yes Minister*. This sharp political satire (and favourite of Mrs Thatcher) starred Paul Eddington as the naive Right Honourable James Hacker, who soon realised that the civil servants ran the government. His adversary was Nigel Hawthorne's Sir Humphrey Appleby, his Permanent Secretary, who always ended up smothering all the minister's

Routledge
Taylor & Francis Group

plans with red tape via long-winded and verbose explanations that the minister could not understand and just accepted. Hawthorne won best comedy BAFTA four times in a row for this character.

Other debuts this year included the consumer complaints show *Watchdog*, presented by Hugh Scully, and the game show *Play Your Cards Right*, hosted by Bruce Forsyth. Here contestants had to guess whether playing card values would be higher or lower than the last one turned over. The audience would shout out 'higher' or 'lower' to sway the contestants.

A record British television audience was reached this year when the James Bond film *Live and Let Die* starring Roger Moore was shown and enjoyed by 23.5 million viewers. Violet Carson made her last appearance as Ena Sharples in *Coronation Street*, which was 20 years old this year. The year also saw the first annual BBC 'Children in Need' fundraiser. Finally, in November millions watched Dallas to find out 'who killed JR?' Can you remember?

Screen and page

Peter Sellers died in July. The ex-Goon had starred in many films, using his considerable comedic talents. Perhaps his most famous role was as Inspector Clouseau in the *Pink Panther* series. His other films included *Dr Strangelove* and *Being There*. An early film, *The Millionairess*, had him playing an Indian doctor with Sophia Loren and a promotional single had him duetting with her on the song *Goodness Gracious Me!* Master of suspense the director Alfred Hitchcock also died this year. How many of his films can you name?

The year's popular film releases included:

The Shining	Jack Nicholson and Shelley Duvall
Star Wars: The Empire Strikes Back	Mark Hamill, Harrison Ford and Carrie Fisher
The Blues Brothers	John Belushi and Dan Ackroyd
Fame	Irene Cara
Raging Bull	Robert De Niro

Routledge
Taylor & Francis Group

Airplane	Leslie Nielsen
The Elephant Man	John Hurt
The Long Riders	David Carradine

In literature, William Golding's novel *Rites of Passage* won the Booker Prize. It was the first part of his 'To the Ends of the Earth' trilogy. Also published this year were *Smiley's People* by John Le Carré, *Midnight's Children* by Salman Rushdie, *The Bourne Identity* by Robert Ludlum and *The Name of the Rose* by Umberto Eco.

Sport

The Winter Olympics were held at Lake Placid, New York and Great Britain's Robin Cousins won a gold medal for figure skating. At the Moscow summer Olympics, Great Britain and Northern Ireland did considerably better, winning 21 medals including five golds. Allan Wells won the 100 metres, Daley Thompson the decathlon and Duncan Goodhew the 100 metres breaststroke. There were two classic showdowns between Steve Ovett and Sebastian Coe. These ended honours even with Ovett winning the 800 metres (Coe came second) and Coe winning the 1500 metres. Sixty-five countries including the USA boycotted the games because of the Soviet war in Afghanistan, which probably explains why we won so many medals that year!

Bjorn Borg won his fifth consecutive Wimbledon title after a mammoth and classic 55-game match against John McEnroe, which included a tie break 23 minutes long.

In football, Liverpool won the Football League for the 12th time. Second Division West Ham beat Arsenal 1–0 in the FA Cup with a Trevor Brooking goal, and in Europe Nottingham Forest retained the European Cup, beating Hamburg SV 1–0.

Routledge
Taylor & Francis Group

Do you remember?

'Jam sandwich' police cars came in this year to replace the old Panda cars, so called because they had a white middle like a panda. The jam sandwich was so named because it was white with a red stripe all the way around! The police had a 45 per cent pay rise in 1979 after Mrs Thatcher came to power and they were to earn their pay in the increasingly volatile inner cities of the early 1980s. Policing became more confrontational under Mrs Thatcher with people being stopped on suspicion under the notorious 'sus' laws, which were to antagonise black youths who were their main victims. Later, in the mid-1980s, the police were to become crucial for the government as they did battle with the trades unions, in particular the miners under Arthur Scargill.

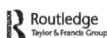 Routledge
Taylor & Francis Group

1980 Personal and local events

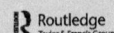

Routledge
Taylor & Francis Group

1981

Major events

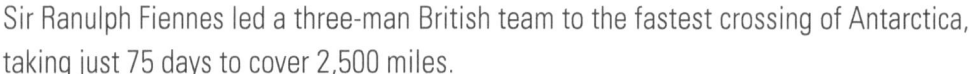

January

Peter Sutcliffe, a 35-year-old Bradford lorry driver, was arrested and later pleaded guilty to 13 'Yorkshire Ripper' murders.

Sir Ranulph Fiennes led a three-man British team to the fastest crossing of Antarctica, taking just 75 days to cover 2,500 miles.

The 52 US Embassy hostages in Iran were released after their 444-day ordeal.

MPs Shirley Williams, Roy Jenkins, William Rodgers and David Owen announced they were to split from the Labour Party and form their own Social Democratic Party.

The government poured £9 billion-worth of aid into ailing motor company British Leyland.

Ronald Reagan was inaugurated as US President.

February

Rock and Roller Bill Hayley died.

The Times newspaper, which had been battling the unions over the introduction of new printing technology and had been forced to shut down for a year, was sold to the Australian Rupert Murdoch.

The Palace announced the engagement of the Prince of Wales to Lady Diana Spencer.

March

The first Homebase DIY and garden superstore opened in Croydon.

The government's Budget announced more public spending cuts. Unemployment was just under 2.5 million, which was around 10 per cent of the workforce.

Nearly 7,000 runners took part in the first London Marathon.

President Reagan was shot in an assassination attempt.

Routledge
Taylor & Francis Group

April

Bobby Sands, an IRA member on hunger strike in the Maze Prison, was elected as a Member of Parliament.

Riots broke out in Brixton, London, an area of high unemployment.

May

Bobby Sands became the first IRA hunger striker to die in the Maze Prison, triggering riots.

Ken Livingstone was elected leader of the Greater London Council.

Pope John Paul II was seriously wounded by a gunman in St Peter's Square, Rome.

Peter Sutcliffe was found guilty of the Yorkshire Ripper murders and later sentenced to life imprisonment.

The TUC's 'March for Jobs' saw 100,000-plus march from across Britain to Trafalgar Square.

June

National Front skinheads clashed with black people in Coventry.

July

Riots and clashes with police occurred in socially deprived areas of London, Liverpool and many other UK inner cities and towns. In Liverpool's Toxteth area the police used CS gas for the first time in mainland Britain. In the ensuing days and weeks rioting spread to many other towns. In Manchester's Moss Side the local police station was besieged and shops were extensively looted.

Mrs Thatcher announced that the police could use rubber bullets and water cannons against rioters.

The Humber Bridge was officially opened by the Queen. At 1,410 metres it was the longest single-span bridge in the world.

Rugby fans clashed with anti-apartheid demonstrators in New Zealand as South Africa's Springboks undertook a controversial tour.

Prince Charles married Lady Diana Spencer, watched by around 700 million people worldwide. In the UK it was a public holiday. In celebration there was a chain of 102

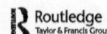

beacons across the British Isles. All sorts of weird and wonderful merchandise appeared everywhere, such as mugs with Charles 'ear' handles, and royal waving hands for car windows as well as the usual biscuits and commemorative paraphernalia … it was hard to get away from the wedding.

August

A million Solidarity members went on strike against food shortages and the economic crisis in Poland.

Moira Stewart became the BBC's first black newsreader.

September

Petrol stations began selling fuel in litres.

The Greenham Common women's peace camp was set up. A group of Welsh women had marched there from Cardiff and when their request for a debate was denied they set up camp. It quickly became a national issue and gained international renown for a campaign which was to last 19 more years.

October

President Sadat was assassinated in Egypt and was succeeded by Hosni Mubarak.

November

Television licence fees increased to £46 for colour and £15 for a black and white set.

A report into the year's riots blamed social and economic problems for the unrest.

December

Arthur Scargill became leader of the National Union of Mineworkers.

The Polish trade union Solidarity was banned after calling for a referendum to oust the government.

Sixteen crew members of the Penlee lifeboat *Solomon Browne*, and the merchant vessel she was sent to rescue, *Union Star*, perished in stormy Cornish seas.

Also this year … the Aids virus was officially recognised and the 'safe sex' message was to become a dominant health theme throughout the 1980s.

On the home front

The term 'yuppy' came into use, meaning 'young urban professional'. These were single, high-earning, middle class over-20s. Bar codes on packaging were increasingly being used as checkouts became more sophisticated, and jogging was becoming increasingly popular. It was often done while listening to music with the new must-have Sony Walkman. Exercise and dance were both coming back into prominence thanks to films such as *Saturday Night Fever* and *Fame*. Combining exercise and dance and boosting the sale of leggings was Olivia Newton John with the song *Physical* ('Let's get into physical. Let me hear your body talk')! This was the best-selling song in the USA and got to number seven in the UK. The accompanying 'raunchy' video showed how far Newton John had come since her 1971 *Banks of the Ohio* country music days. The video also heralded a move towards much more 'steamy' videos and underlined the modern importance of the video for selling the music. Some would say that many videos were better than the songs! Such developments could only mean one thing … Madonna was waiting in the wings!

Music

Can you recall these lyrics: 'Don't you ever, don't you ever, stop being dandy, showing me you're handsome'? They were from *Prince Charming* by Adam and the Ants, who were very big in 1981. Bucks Fizz were to become big too as they won the Eurovision Song Contest with *Making Your Mind Up.*

Other popular singles included:

Tainted Love	Soft Cell
This Ole House	Shakin' Stevens
Vienna	Ultravox
The Birdie Song	The Tweets
Ghost Town	The Specials
Don't You Want Me?	The Human League
Body Talk	Imagination
In the Air Tonight	Phil Collins
Every Little Thing She Does is Magic	The Police

Television

Tom Baker left *Dr Who* after seven years in the role, to be replaced by Peter Davidson. Two days before the Royal Wedding, *Coronation Street* staged its own high-profile wedding as Ken Barlow and Deirdre Langton tied the knot.

Debuts this year included:

Only Fools and Horses. This starred David Jason as Del Boy Trotter and Nicholas Lyndhurst as Rodney … 'You plonker!' The series followed the adventures and disasters of the Peckham black market wheeler-dealers and market traders as they sought to become millionaires. They drove a yellow Robin Reliant emblazoned with the logo 'Trotters Independent Trading'! They lived in a high-rise council flat in Nelson Mandela House with Grandad. Their regular colleagues were the hapless Trigger and the used car salesman Boycie. It was destined to become one of the UK's most popular sitcoms.

Other debuts this year included *Postman Pat,* the television adaptation of Evelyn Waugh's novel *Brideshead Revisited, Bergerac* with John Nettles and *Game for a Laugh.* Also popular was the zany comedian Kenny Everett, whose catchphrase was 'It's all in the best possible taste'.

Screen and page

This year's film releases included:

The French Lieutenant's Woman	Meryl Streep
Raiders of the Lost Ark	Harrison Ford
Das Boot	Jürgen Prochnow
Time Bandits	David Rappaport
An American Werewolf in London	David Naughton
For Your Eyes Only	Roger Moore
Reds	Warren Beatty and Diane Keaton
Escape to Victory	Michael Caine, Pele, Bobby Moore, Sylvester Stallone

Routledge
Taylor & Francis Group

On Golden Pond	Henry Fonda and Katherine Hepburn
Gregory's Girl	John Gordon Sinclair
Gallipoli	Mel Gibson

This year publications included *Rabbit is Rich* by John Updike, *Sharp's Eagle* by Bernard Cornwell, *The Hotel New Hampshire* by John Irving and *The Mosquito Coast* by Paul Theroux.

Sport

Liverpool won the European Cup for the third time, beating Real Madrid 1–0. Sadness was to hit the club later in the year though, when the legendary manager Bill Shankly died aged 67.

See if you can answer these sporting questions:

Who won the World Snooker Championship aged 23?   *Steve Davis*

The Aga Khan's horse won the Derby, the Irish Derby, the King George VI and Queen Elizabeth stakes – what was its name?   *Shergar*

Jockey Bob Champion, a cancer survivor, won the Grand National on which horse? *Aldaniti*

Who threw several tantrums as he became the new Wimbledon men's champion, beating Bjorn Borg, who he had lost to the previous year?   *John McEnroe*

This year's FA Cup was the 100th and was taken to a replay with which team eventually beating Manchester City 3–2?   *Tottenham Hotspur*

Who became Britain's most expensive player when West Bromwich Albion sold him to Manchester United for £1.5 million?   *Bryan Robson*

England qualified for the World Cup by beating which country 1–0? It was the first time they had qualified since 1970.   *Hungary*

Which pair won the European and World Figure Skating Championships?   *Jayne Torvill and Christopher Dean*

Do you remember?

Beginning in 1971 but still at the height of their popularity were the two Ronnies, Corbett and Barker. Their sketch show had them as newsreaders swapping one-liners and clever word play. Famous sketches included 'Four candles/fork handles' and a version of *Mastermind* where Corbett would give the right answer, but to the previous question. Corbett would also do meandering monologues sitting in his chair facing the camera. As with Morecambe and Wise there would always be a musical finale, and the show ended back with the newsreaders and the final line, 'It's goodnight from me, and it's goodnight from him, goodnight'.

1981 Personal and local events

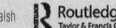

1982

Major events

January
The UK recorded its lowest-ever temperature at minus 27.2 degrees C in Braemar, Aberdeenshire.

Miners accepted a 9.6 per cent pay offer and averted a strike.

Unemployment topped three million.

Rioting broke out in the St Pauls district of Bristol.

February
Sir Freddie Laker's Laker Airways went bust, stranding 6,000 passengers.

Clothing stores Hepworths and Kendalls merged to form Next.

March
The last steam-driven weaving mill in Burnley closed.

Argentinian troops landed on South Georgia, a British overseas territory.

April
Argentinian troops invaded the Falkland Islands and overthrew the British administration, starting the Falklands War. The islands had been a British colony for over 150 years. The Royal Navy sent a task force and Britain announced a 200-mile exclusion zone around the islands.

Twenty-three days later, Royal Marines recaptured South Georgia.

May
A Vulcan bomber took off from Ascension Island and bombed Port Stanley airport to prevent the Argentinians using it to land troops and supplies.

The Argentinian cruiser *General Belgrano* was sunk by a British submarine, killing around 360. Two days later *HMS Sheffield* was sunk by Exocet missiles.

Routledge
Taylor & Francis Group

Kielder Water reservoir, the largest artificial lake in the UK, was opened. It was surrounded by the largest planted woodland in Europe.

Pope John Paul II visited Britain and attended an Anglican service at Canterbury Cathedral.

June

Argentinian forces surrendered as British troops reached Port Stanley after having 'yomped' across the island. General Galtieri resigned as President of Argentina.

Prince William was born on the 21st.

July

An intruder at Buckingham Palace got into the Queen's bedroom and chatted to her before he was apprehended.

Eight soldiers and seven horses were killed as IRA bombs packed with nails exploded in London's Hyde Park and Regent's Park. The horses were part of the Household Cavalry making their way to the changing of the guard. In Regent's Park the bomb was detonated under a bandstand where an army band was playing.

September

Former Hollywood star Princess Grace of Monaco died in a car crash aged 52. She was thought to have suffered a stroke at the wheel and driven off a mountain pass. Her younger daughter, Stephanie, survived the crash and went on to become a fashion model.

Figures showed that around 14 per cent of the workforce were unemployed, but the government changed the way the statistics were collected, counting only those who were claiming benefit rather than those registered as unemployed, thus making the picture look brighter than it was.

October

The *Mary Rose*, Henry VIII's flagship built in 1545, was raised from the seabed in the Solent. It had spent 437 years on the seabed and was on its way to engage the French when it mysteriously sank.

Halley's Comet was seen for the first time since 1911.

Routledge
Taylor & Francis Group

November

Channel 4 went on air.

December

Thousands of women linked hands and encircled the nine-mile perimeter fence of Greenham Common airbase in protest at the siting there of US nuclear Cruise missiles.

Also this year … Jane Fonda released the first of her exercise videos, *Jane Fonda's Workout.* It became one of the highest-selling videos over the next few years and, following on from the previous year's London Marathon, there was a gym and fitness boom.

On the home front

Well over 50 per cent of households now had their own telephones. In the kitchen, microwaves were giving us meals in minutes and there were ever-increasing varieties of processed, easy-to-cook and frozen meals available. However, there was still a great interest in cookery, as witnessed by the success of the television show *Madhur Jaffrey's Indian Cookery*, which urged us to experiment with spices. In contrast to this, television cook Anton Mosimann was extolling the virtues of 'nouvelle cuisine', where the emphasis was on lighter cooking and fancy presentation. It was cynically referred to as 'posh nosh'! At the same time, the Chinese cook Ken Hom was becoming very popular, triggering a boom in wok sales. Buying the ingredients was becoming ever-more reliant on having your own transport as supermarkets were increasingly moving out of town centres.

This year saw the launch of the modern-looking Ford Sierra, replacing the more conventional Cortina, which had been around for years. For those too young to drive, BMX bikes were very popular.

Music

The year's best-selling singles included:

It Ain't What You Do
It's The Way That You Do It   Bananarama

Do You Really Want To Hurt Me?	Culture Club
Rio	Duran Duran
Come on Eileen	Dexy's Midnight Runners
Fame	Irene Cara
Eye of the Tiger	Survivor
The Lion Sleeps Tonight	Tight Fit
I Don't Wanna Dance	Eddy Grant
Ebony and Ivory	Paul McCartney and Stevie Wonder
Town Called Malice	The Jam
Love Plus One	Haircut One Hundred
House of Fun	Madness
Pass the Dutchie	Musical Youth

Television

Channel 4 began broadcasting this year. Its first programme was *Countdown* with Richard Whiteley. One of its other early favourite programmes was the soap opera *Brookside*. The channel also debuted its innovative music programme *The Tube* hosted by Jools Holland and Jessica Yates.

One drama series often cited by many as evocative of the decade was Alan Bleasdale's *Boys from the Blackstuff* starring Bernard Hill as Yosser Hughes. It was the story of five unemployed Liverpudlian men and was a dramatic commentary on the 'Thatcher years'. Critical in tone, it depicted the social and psychological impact of unemployment on the men and their families. Yosser's catchphrases were 'Gis a job' and 'I can do that'. It was both sad and funny at the same time.

Television debuts included *Dynasty* as a rival to *Dallas*, the chat show *Wogan*, the history and archaeology programme *Timewatch* and the comedy *The Young Ones* with Rik Mayall, Adrian Edmondson, Nigel Planer and Alexei Sayle. This slightly anarchic series brought alternative comedy to the small screen and was a sign of things to come.

Routledge Taylor & Francis Group

Back in mainstream comedy but no less funny was the clever wartime series *'Allo, 'Allo.* 'Listen very carefully, I shall say this only once'! The show was set in Nazi-occupied France in the café of René Artois, played by Gordon Kaye. He was assisted by his domineering wife Edith, 'you stupid woman', and his waitress Yvette who was in love with him. Other characters included Michelle of the Resistance, Monsieur 'it is I, LeClerc' LeClerc, General von Klinkerhoffen, Herr Flick of the Gestapo and two bumbling English airmen in hiding. There was also officer Crabtree, an Englishman posing as a French policeman, with a terrible French accent, 'Good Moaning'.

Screen and page

The year's best film releases included *Gandhi*, which went on to win eight Oscars including best actor for Ben Kingsley and best director for Richard Attenborough. Other impressive films were:

E.T. the Extra-Terrestrial	Drew Barrymore
Blade Runner	Harrison Ford
Poltergeist	JoBeth Williams
Tootsie	Dustin Hoffman and Jessica Lange
An Officer and a Gentleman	Richard Gere and Debra Winger
The Wall	Bob Geldof
Sophie's Choice	Meryl Streep and Kevin Kline

In literature, *Schindler's Ark* by Thomas Keneally won the Booker Prize and other worthy publications were *On the Black Hill* by Bruce Chatwin, *The Secret Diary of Adrian Mole, Aged 13¾* by Sue Townsend, *A Mind to Murder* by P. D. James, Alice Walker's *The Color Purple*, *The BFG* by Roald Dahl and *War Horse* by Michael Morpurgo.

Sport

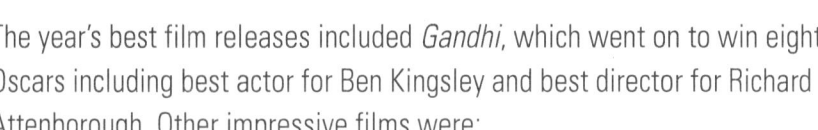

In cricket, several players including Geoff Boycott and Graham Gooch went on a rebel tour of apartheid-ridden South Africa, earning them a three-year Test cricket ban. They were soundly beaten by South Africa. In the European Athletics

Championships Daley Thompson became the first man in any event to hold the Olympic, European and Commonwealth titles as he regained the world decathlon record. And in football, the FA Cup Final was taken to a replay again as Spurs beat Queens Park Rangers 1–0. England were knocked out of the World Cup in the group stages and manager Ron Greenwood retired, to be replaced by Bobby Robson. Italy went on to win the tournament for the third time and Diego Maradona transferred to Barcelona for a record £5 million.

Do you remember?

New Romantics! Culture Club with Boy George were part of what became known as the 'New Romantic' movement, characterised by eccentric dress and flamboyant hairstyles such as the 'mullet'. At its peak in the early 1980s it was partly a reaction against the anti-fashion stance of Punk music. It also tended to be somewhat androgynous, with boys wearing eyeliner and make-up. Padded shoulders were also favoured. Ultravox, Spandau Ballet, Adam and the Ants and The Human League were other contemporary examples. Frilly shirts and eccentricity in dress were partly fuelled by Vivienne Westwood, who was popular at the time and certainly inspired Adam Ant's pirate look. As the music evolved with the rise of the synthesiser sound, so the fashion gradually changed, with sharp suits becoming popular; Duran Duran epitomised this. Along with the fine clothes came finely made videos and Duran Duran hired professional directors to make theirs.

Routledge
Taylor & Francis Group

1982 Personal and local events

Routledge
Taylor & Francis Group

1983

Major events

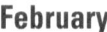

January
The wearing of seatbelts in cars became compulsory.

Red rain fell, caused by sand from the Sahara.

February
Unemployment reached a record high of 3.2 million.

Mass murderer Dennis Nilsen was arrested and subsequently found guilty of killing 15 men over the previous four years. He was subsequently sentenced to life imprisonment.

April
The US Embassy in Beirut was bombed, killing over 30.

The one pound coin was introduced. To make it recognisable it was thicker than other coins and had a yellow colour.

May
Wheel clamps were used for the first time in the UK.

June
With their popularity restored by the victory in the Falklands War, the Conservative Party under Margaret Thatcher was re-elected with a landslide victory on 9 June. It was at this election that Tony Blair and Gordon Brown were first elected to Parliament. The SDP–Liberal Alliance came a poor third. Michael Foot, the Labour leader, resigned several days later, as did the SDP's Roy Jenkins.

July
Hot on the heels of the election, Chancellor Nigel Lawson announced more public spending cuts to the tune of £500 million.

August
New car registration plates were introduced, prefixed with an A.

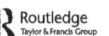

September

The NHS privatised its catering and cleaning service.

Thirty-eight IRA prisoners escaped from the Maze Prison.

October

Neil Kinnock became the leader of the Labour Party.

Lech Walesa was awarded the Nobel Peace Prize.

Over one million joined a CND march in London.

November

Demonstrations at Greenham Common saw many women arrested as the first Cruise missiles arrived.

The Brinks Mat robbery occurred, with crooks getting away with £26 million worth of gold bars from a vault at Heathrow.

December

The first heart and lung transplant in Britain took place at Harefield Hospital.

An IRA bomb at Harrods killed six people on one of the busiest Christmas shopping days. Among the dead were three policemen.

Also this year … recession was a serious concern across the globe, even in the USA and Japan. In the UK, unemployment remained a huge concern, with over 12 per cent of the workforce unable to find jobs. In the Lebanese capital Beirut, war waged all year between opposing factions, reducing the city to a crumbling ruin. Compact discs went on sale in Britain for the first time, heralding the demise of the vinyl LP.

On the home front

'Ghetto blaster' radio and tape players were all the rage as 'cool dudes' swaggered around the streets, annoying others with their favourite tunes. On a cleaner note, the bathtime must-have was a bottle of Matey bubble bath. Shaped like a skittle and looking like a sailor, these bottles were the precursors of all character-shaped bubble bath bottles to come.

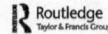

In fashion, the 1980s was the decade of the dreaded mullet hairstyle, as modelled by Kevin Keegan among others. It was also an era of dancing films such as *Flashdance*, *Dirty Dancing* and *Fame*, so we had a resurgence of leggings to complement the huge shoulder pads which by now were a common fashion feature. These were nowhere more in evidence than on the popular US television shows *Dynasty* and *Dallas*. Can you recall the protagonists in these television series? At the Southfork Ranch, *Dallas* had J. R. Ewing, Sue Ellen, Bobby, Pamela and their adversary Cliff Barnes, while *Dynasty* boasted the Carringtons with Blake and Krystle and his ex-wife Alexis played by Joan Collins. 'Power dressing' was the phrase coined to describe the assertive nature of much 1980s fashion. Both Mrs Thatcher and Lady Di used it. For Mrs Thatcher it helped to give her prominence and authority in the very male-dominated world of politics. Her sharp suits with matching shoes and handbags were to represent the equivalent of the male pinstripe three-piece city suit. Lady Diana also helped to popularise powerful clothes with her shoulder pads.

Another mid-1980s fashion fad was the sweatband, popularised by John McEnroe and Mark Knopfler of Dire Straits.

Music

For many, one of the albums of the decade was Michael Jackson's *Thriller*, which became the best-selling album of all time. He was also known for his dancing skills, especially his famous 'Moonwalk'! The accompanying video was a horror spoof with dancing zombies and werewolves. Can you name the artists responsible for these other 1983 albums? *No Parlez*, *Colour by Numbers*, *Labour of Love*, *Rio* and *War*.

The most popular singles of the year included:

Karma Chameleon	Culture Club
Uptown Girl	Billy Joel
Red Red Wine	UB40
Too Shy	Kajagoogoo
Total Eclipse of the Heart	Bonnie Tyler
Billie Jean	Michael Jackson

Routledge Taylor & Francis Group

Sweet Dreams Are Made of This	The Eurythmics
All Night Long	Lionel Ritchie
Wherever I Lay My Hat, That's My Home	Paul Young
Every Breath You Take	The Police
Flashdance ... What a Feeling	Irene Cara

Television

In television, the children's channel CITV was launched, as was the first UK breakfast show, the BBC's *Breakfast Time*, initially presented by Frank Bough, Selina Scott and Nick Ross. It was a strange mixture of news, sport and cosy chat. ITV quickly followed suit with *Good Morning Britain* presented by Anne Diamond and Nick Owen.

This year also gave us the sitcom *Blackadder*, starring Rowan Atkinson and his hapless servant Baldrick, played by Tony Robinson. Also debuting was: 'If you have a problem, if no one can help, and if you can find them, maybe you can hire ...' *The A Team*.

In children's television, we had the teenagers' quiz *Blockbusters*. Its contestants were sixth formers and it was hosted by Bob Holness. You had to answer questions and make your way across a board of hexagons without getting blocked by your opponents, a bit like checkers. Questions were based on letters of the alphabet and a favourite phrase for the young contestants was 'Can I have a P please Bob?'!

In *Coronation Street*, millions watched Deirdre leave Mike Baldwin to go back to Ken Barlow! This year also saw the actor Peter Adamson last play Len Fairclough in the series and Doris Speed step down as Annie Walker, the landlady of the Rovers Return. *Dr Who* was 20 years old this year and was played by Peter Davidson, the fifth Doctor. Can you name his four predecessors? Going backwards in time they were Tom Baker, John Pertwee, Patrick Troughton and the first Doctor, William Hartnell. For many, however, the best comedy drama on television this year was *Auf Wiedersehen Pet*, the story of the shenanigans of British building workers in Germany.

Routledge
Taylor & Francis Group

Screen and page

A great British film appeared this year, *Educating Rita,* starring Michael Caine and Julie Walters. It told of the unlikely platonic relationship between Caine's alcoholic university professor and Walters' working class Liverpudlian housewife trying to better herself by studying literature.

Other popular films released this year included:

Star Wars: Return of the Jedi	Mark Hamill, Carrie Fisher, Harrison Ford
Trading Places	Eddie Murphy and Dan Ackroyd
Octopussy	Roger Moore and Maud Adams
Never Say Never Again	Sean Connery and Kim Basinger
Flashdance	Jennifer Beals
The Meaning of Life	The *Monty Python* cast
Merry Christmas Mr Lawrence	David Bowie and Tom Conti
Local Hero	Burt Lancaster and Fulton Mackay

July 29 saw the death of actor David Niven. Can you name some of his films? Here's just a few: *A Matter of Life and Death*, *The Pink Panther*, *The Elusive Pimpernel* and *The Guns of Navarone.*

In the world of books, William Golding won the Nobel Prize for Literature. It has been said that his novels 'illuminated the human condition in the world today'. The year's best published works included *The Colour of Magic* by Terry Pratchett, the first in his 'Discworld' series, *The Mists of Avalon* by M. Z. Bradley, *Babe: The Gallant Pig* by Dick King Smith and *Hollywood Wives* by Jackie Collins.

Sport

The four-yearly Athletics World Championships were inaugurated. The first one, in Helsinki, saw Carl Lewis take gold in the long jump and 100 metres. Steve Cram won the 1,500 metres and Daley Thompson won the decathlon.

 Routledge
Taylor & Francis Group

Pat Jennings, the Arsenal and Northern Ireland goalkeeper, played his 1,000th senior game, the first player to do so. He had his longest spell with London rivals Spurs.

Manchester United beat Brighton and Hove Albion 4–0 in the FA Cup, which once again had to go to a replay after an initial 2–2 draw.

Seve Ballesteros won his second green jacket at the US Open in Augusta.

Do you remember?

Duran Duran! They were one of the most successful New Romantic bands of the 1980s. Their early use of 'raunchy' videos coincided with the new US music channel MTV, and this helped to propel them to fame as the better videos got shown more often. However, they also had some very good songs, such as *Hungry Like the Wolf*, *Save a Prayer*, *Rio*, *Is There Something I Should Know* and *The Reflex*. In 1985 they went on to do the theme tune to the James Bond film *A View To Kill*, cementing their reputation. They were Simon Le Bon, Nick Rhodes, Andy Taylor, Roger Taylor and John Taylor.

Routledge
Taylor & Francis Group

1983 Personal and local events

1984

Major events

January

George Orwell's 1984 vision wasn't quite as bad as the book!

Six died as hurricane force winds hit Britain.

February

US astronauts became the first to walk in space untethered.

The Winter Olympics began in Sarajevo and a week later skaters Jayne Torvill and Christopher Dean took the gold medal for ice dancing to Ravel's *Bolero*.

March

The dockyards at Chatham closed. Ships had been built there since the reign of Henry VIII.

Miners in the UK went on strike against layoffs and plans to close many pits. The strike was to last a year.

French farmers were protesting about foreign meat imports. They hijacked and burnt lorries carrying meat from other EEC member states.

April

This month saw the start of many clashes between striking miners and police. Miners' leader Arthur Scargill ruled out the possibility of a ballot.

Comedian Tommy Cooper collapsed from a heart attack and died on stage.

Policewoman Yvonne Fletcher was killed by a gunman firing from the Libyan Embassy in London. Britain severed diplomatic relations with Libya.

May

The Thames Barrier was opened by the Queen. Its purpose was to protect London from tidal surges.

Routledge
Taylor & Francis Group

Poet Laureate John Betjeman died.

Orgreave Colliery was the scene of fierce clashes between police and miners. Arthur Scargill was arrested and charged with obstruction.

June

It was announced that O levels and CSEs were to be replaced by GCSEs over the next few years.

York Minster was struck by lightning and the ensuing blaze was fought by 150 firefighters. The 13th-century south transept roof was destroyed and the 16th-century stained glass rose window was damaged. It cost £2.25 million to painstakingly repair over the next four years.

Robert Maxwell bought the *Daily Mirror*.

The government brought in the Trades Union Act, which outlawed strikes without a ballot.

September

Fourteen people were killed in rioting in Sharpeville, South Africa, while protesting at racist legislation.

The Princess of Wales gave birth to Prince Harry.

October

Five people died when the IRA bombed the Grand Hotel in Brighton, where most of the Conservative Cabinet were staying during their annual conference.

BBC newsreader Michael Buerk described the terrible famine in Ethiopia which was to spark the Feed the World campaign and Live Aid.

Indian Prime Minister Indira Gandhi was assassinated by two Sikhs. Over 1,000 died in the riots that ensued as Hindu mobs sought revenge on the Sikh community.

November

Ronald Reagan was re-elected as US President.

The one pound note was withdrawn from circulation.

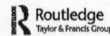

British Telecom shares went on sale. This was very popular, with almost 5 per cent of the population buying shares.

Pop musicians formed Band Aid and recorded the song *Do They Know It's Christmas?* to raise money for Ethiopian famine relief.

December
A toxic gas leak killed thousands in Bhopal, India.

Also this year … famine ravaged many African countries, with Ethiopia being hit the worst. More than a million people died of starvation during the year and a graphic BBC news report showed a child dying on camera. An international relief effort was set up but was hampered by wars and poor transport networks.

On the home front

This was obviously the decade of the shoulder pad and bringing it to menswear was the television series *Miami Vice* with US actor Don Johnson making the expensive jacket and T-shirt combo all the rage. For the full fashion effect you had to roll up the jacket sleeves. Political slogans on T-shirts were all the rage too, popularised by designer Katherine Hamnett, and many took to broadcasting such messages as 'Save the future' and 'Ban pollution'. Hamnett wore one saying '58 per cent don't want Pershing' when she met Prime Minister Margaret Thatcher. Many were opposed to the US Pershing missiles being based in the UK.

In the office, Filofaxes were becoming the must-have item. These spiral-bound diaries and organisers were all the rage with upwardly mobile yuppies and city business workers. In the home, at a time when the UK population was 56.4 million we had 23 million television sets and so most households would have had one by now. Can you remember these two shows?

Treasure Hunt. Anneka Rice in a jumpsuit rushed between locations in a helicopter against the clock, following the directions of a studio team who were trying to work out clues as to the whereabouts of some treasure. She would leap out of the helicopter and startle some unsuspecting member of the public by asking them directions to a local landmark.

The Krypton Factor, presented by Gordon Burns, was a quiz show involving both mental and physical challenges. Rounds included watching a short film and then being tested on your powers of observation, assault courses and three-dimensional puzzles to solve and put together.

Music

In November, Bob Geldof of the Boomtown Rats and Midge Ure of Ultravox bought many top pop musicians together to record the chart topping single *Do They Know It's Christmas?* in aid of Ethiopian famine relief. Music was a big issue this year even before Bob Geldof began to mobilise forces for Band Aid. The duo Wham were hugely popular. George Michael and Andrew Ridgeley sported permed hair, shoulder padded jackets with rolled-up sleeves and T-shirts with slogans such as 'Choose Life'! Their 1984 single *Last Christmas* has become one of the Christmas songs we hear every year. However, it only got to number two in the charts because it was pipped by Band Aid's *Do They Know It's Christmas?* Wham split in 1986 but George Michael went on to achieve superstardom. This year was also responsible for what may well be the worst song of the decade, *Agadoo* by Black Lace. It is hard to get out of your mind once you recall it. Played at many a disco, it conjurs up images of elderly relatives at weddings, a bit worse the wear for drink and making an exhibition of themselves doing a conga around the dance floor. The only other song which comes close to qualifying is *The Birdie Song* by The Tweets!

This year's other popular singles included:

Wake Me Up Before You Go Go	Wham
Purple Rain	Prince
Holiday	Madonna
I Just Called To Say I Love You	Stevie Wonder
Relax	Frankie Goes to Hollywood
Pride (In the Name of Love)	U2
Agadoo	Black Lace
What's Love Got To Do With It	Tina Turner

Routledge
Taylor & Francis Group

I Want To Break Free	Queen
Girls Just Want To Have Fun	Cyndi Lauper

Can you recall who recorded these albums?

Alf	Alison Moyet
Welcome to the Pleasuredome	Frankie Goes to Hollywood
The Unforgettable Fire	U2
Born in the USA	Bruce Springsteen

Television

Spitting Image, with its unique blend of latex puppets and satire, began this year. It had great fun with politicians, especially Margaret Thatcher portrayed as a demonic psychopath. Other debuts this year included *Crimewatch*, originally presented by Nick Ross and Sue Cook, who was replaced a year later by Jill Dando. Also new to our screens was *Alas Smith and Jones*, *The Bill* and *The Price is Right*, hosted by Leslie Crowther with his catchphrase 'Come on down!' *Surprise Surprise* with Cilla Black also began; in this show Cilla would surprise people by reuniting them with long-lost friends and relatives or making their dreams come true. This year also gave us *The Jewel in the Crown*, a popular drama series about the last days of the British Raj in India. It starred Art Malik, Charles Dance, Peggy Ashcroft and Geraldine James. In children's television, *Thomas the Tank Engine* came to the screen, narrated by Beatle Ringo Starr, and Peter Davidson made his last appearance as Dr Who when he morphed into Colin Baker. Back in the real world, David Attenborough's *The Living Planet* was a follow-up to his very popular *Life on Earth* series.

Screen and page

John Betjeman, the Poet Laureate, died on 19 April. He loved the English countryside and its traditions and churches. He was replaced as Poet Laureate by Ted Hughes. Another England-loving author, dramatist and broadcaster, J. B. Priestley, died aged 89.

Notable publications this year included Milan Kundera's *The Unbearable Lightness of Being*, J. G. Ballard's *The Empire of the Sun*, Iain Banks's *The Wasp Factory*, Anita Brookner's *Hotel du Lac* and *Flaubert's Parrot* by Julian Barnes.

Anthony Sher caused a sensation in the theatre with his interpretation of *Richard III*.

In film, Welsh actor Richard Burton died this year aged 58. Famous for his romances and marriages to Elizabeth Taylor, his many roles included *Cleopatra*, *Equus*, *Where Eagles Dare*, *The Sandpiper*, *Look Back in Anger*, *Under Milk Wood*, *The Desert Rats* and *The Robe*.

James Mason also died, aged 75. An English actor who made the transition to Hollywood, he made over 120 films including *Lolita*, *The Wicked Lady*, *20,000 Leagues Under the Sea*, *Journey to the Centre of the Earth* and *North by Northwest*.

Popular films released this year included:

A Passage to India	Victor Banerjee and Peggy Ashcroft
Indiana Jones and the Temple of Doom	Harrison Ford
A Nightmare on Elm Street	Johnny Depp
The Terminator	Arnold Schwarzenegger
Ghostbusters	Bill Murphy, Dan Ackroyd and Sigourney Weaver
Gremlins	Zach Galligan and Phoebe Cates
The Killing Fields	Sam Waterstone

Sport

Great Britain and Northern Ireland won five gold medals at the Olympics in Los Angeles. Sebastian Coe won the 1,500 metres, Daley Thompson the decathlon and Tessa Sanderson the women's javelin. South African athlete Zola Budd joined the British Olympic team after a campaign to get her a British passport to overcome the ban on South African athletes. She famously used to run barefoot and collided with the American Mary Decker in the 3,000 metres, putting both out of the medals. American athlete Carl Lewis won four gold medals. Fourteen Eastern Bloc countries boycotted the

Routledge
Taylor & Francis Group

games in response to the US boycott four years previously when the games were held in Moscow. In the Winter Olympics at Sarajevo, Torvill and Dean achieved 12 perfect scores for artistic impression and won the gold medal in free ice dancing.

Darts on television was very popular and darts player John Lowe was at his peak as he recorded the first televised nine-dart finish. Meanwhile, as John McEnroe won his third Wimbledon title, Martina Navratilova won the French Open, the US Open and her fifth Wimbledon title!

Everton won the FA Cup, beating Watford 2–0, and Liverpool won the European Cup for the fourth time, beating AS Roma after a penalty shoot-out. They also won the First Division Championship and the League Cup!

Do you remember?

My Little Pony! These were just getting to be a big craze. The tiny, garish, pastel coloured, doe-eyed, beribboned plastic ponies with long flowing manes and tails were a huge hit with little girls the world over. They came with a raft of plastic (mostly pink) accessories such as their own carriages and castles to live in – a sort of Cinderella world for ponies. They all had babyish names such as Snuzzle and Cotton Candy.

Routledge
Taylor & Francis Group

1984 Personal and local events

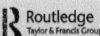

Routledge
Taylor & Francis Group

1985

Major events

January

The first mobile phone call in the UK was made by comedian Ernie Wise.

British inventor Clive Sinclair launched his electric vehicle, the C5. Supposedly running on a washing machine motor and likened by some to driving a shoe, it could only travel at 15 mph. It never caught on!

BT announced it was to phase out red telephone boxes.

March

UK coalminers ended their year-long strike.

Soviet premier Konstantin Chernenko died and was succeeded by Mikhail Gorbachev. It was to be Gorbachev who helped to bring Russia closer to the West, and gave us the words *perestroika*, meaning restructuring, and *glasnost*, meaning openness.

Mohamed Al-Fayed bought Harrods.

April

Israel began withdrawal from Lebanon.

Bernie Grant became the first black council leader when he was elected in Haringey.

May

A fire under a wooden stand at Bradford City Football Club killed 56 people as they watched a match against Lincoln City. A cigarette butt had set light to accumulated rubbish underneath the stand.

Forty-one people died at Heysel Stadium in Brussels as UK soccer hooligans rioted at the European Cup Final between Juventus and Liverpool. As a result UK football clubs were banned from Europe indefinitely.

July

Thirteen-year-old Ruth Lawrence gained a First in Mathematics from Oxford to become its youngest-ever graduate.

Greenpeace ship *Rainbow Warrior* was blown up in New Zealand by French agents. The crew were protesting about nearby French nuclear tests.

Live Aid concerts in London and Philadelphia were watched by over 1.5 billion in 152 countries and raised £70 million-plus in aid of Ethiopian famine victims.

August

Fifty-five were killed when a Boeing 737 bound for Corfu burst into flames on the runway at Manchester airport.

September

The wreck of the *Titanic* was located.

Rioting in Birmingham reignited racial tensions.

Around 20,000 died in a massive earthquake in Mexico City.

October

A report into the Toxteth riots by Lord Scarman blamed economic deprivation and racial discrimination.

Cynthia Jarrett, a black woman, died in police custody after falling down, sparking the Broadwater Farm riots in which PC Keith Blakelock was fatally stabbed.

November

A volcanic eruption in Columbia claimed the lives of around 25,000 as a vast area was covered in a sea of mud.

British Home Stores and Habitat merged.

December

The charity Comic Relief was launched.

Also this year … the hole in the ozone layer over the Antarctic was discovered by the British Antarctic Survey.

Routledge
Taylor & Francis Group

On the home front

Must-have toys included Transformers, based on Japanese comic book characters. They were robots who could change into cars, boats, planes, guns and so on. When you twisted them around they transformed into their other form. Their popularity was ensured as the cartoon series was on television at the same time.

Many women were exercising in front of their television screen to *Jane Fonda's Workout* fitness videos, complete with leotard, leggings and headband. *BBC Breakfast* had the 'Green Goddess' Diane Moran in her shiny green leotard putting the nation through its paces early in the morning. A fashion disaster of the 1980s was the garish shellsuit, as worn by many a young person.

Woolworths was still a big name on the high street, but more shops were moving to big shopping malls and the larger branches of 'Woolies' were disappearing. Huge supermarkets with plenty of parking sold almost all you would need, from groceries to clothes and kitchen appliances, putting a great deal of pressure on small retailers who could not buy in bulk and so were undercut by the larger shops. But what did things cost the shopper in 1985? The following are approximate prices:

Loaf of bread	50p
Milk	22p a pint
Leather shoes	£15 plus
Whisky	£7 a bottle, 65p a shot in the pub
Beer	80p a pint
Wine	£2 a bottle, 65p a glass in the pub
Eggs	80p a dozen
2 lbs (1 kg) potatoes	10p
1 lb (0.5 kg) bacon	£1.40
Large tin of beans	55p
Packet of cornflakes	92p

Routledge
Taylor & Francis Group

1 lb Cheddar cheese	£1.30
Cadbury's Flake	18p
1 apple	10p
2 lbs sugar	47p
10 fish fingers	85p

The average price of a three-bedroom semi was £30,000 and a family car was anything between £5,000 and £8,000.

Gardening and Do It Yourself were popular hobbies and huge DIY stores such as B&Q were springing up all over, just like the out-of-town supermarkets. They often had garden centres attached and such superstores heralded the demise of local family-run ironmonger's shops.

Music

Brothers in Arms by Dire Straits becomes the first million-selling CD.

Best-selling singles this year included:

The Power of Love	Jennifer Rush
Into the Groove	Madonna
Dancing in the Street	David Bowie and Mick Jagger
I Want To Know What Love Is	Foreigner
I'm Your Man	Wham
Everybody Wants to Rule the World	Tears for Fears
Dancing in the Dark	Bruce Springsteen
Money for Nothing	Dire Straits
That Ole Devil Called Love	Alison Moyet
Saving All My Love For You	Whitney Houston

Ⓡ Routledge
Taylor & Francis Group

Television

On 19 February *EastEnders* was broadcast for the first time. It was destined to become a hugely popular rival to *Coronation Street*. Set in Albert Square in the fictional East End borough of Walford, its characters included the Beale and Fowler families and of course the landlady of the Queen Vic, Angie, her husband 'Dirty' Den and their daughter Sharon. They were soon to be joined by such characters as Dot Cotton, Pat Wicks (Pat Butcher) and later the Mitchell family. Another debut this year was *Blind Date* with Cilla Black. Here a contestant chose a member of the opposite sex based on their answers to questions and the couple were sent on a date. They then returned to tell all about how it went.

The world of alternative comedy was also brought to our screen with *Saturday Live*. Hosted by stand-up comedian Ben Elton, it also starred Harry Enfield, whose memorable personas included Stavros, who ran a Greek restaurant, and the nauseating Cockney plasterer Loadsamoney. It also featured Stephen Fry, Hugh Laurie, Adrian Edmondson and Rik Mayall.

Screen and page

Three famous actors died this year: Rock Hudson (59), Orson Welles (60) and Yul Brynner (65). Compiling a list of their respective movies will bring back many memories. Here are some, but can you remember who starred in which?

The King and I	Yul Brynner (with Deborah Kerr)
Citizen Kane	Orson Welles
Magnificent Obsession	Rock Hudson (with Jane Wyman)
The Third Man	Orson Welles
The Magnificent Seven	Yul Brynner (with Eli Wallach, Steve McQueen, Charles Bronson, Robert Vaughan, Brad Dexter, and James Coburn)
A Farewell to Arms	Rock Hudson (with Jennifer Jones)
Westworld	Yul Brynner

Routledge
Taylor & Francis Group

Touch of Evil	Orson Welles
Pillow Talk	Rock Hudson (with Doris Day)
Solomon and Sheba	Yul Brynner (with Gina Lollobrigida)
Tobruk	Rock Hudson
The Lady from Shanghai	Orson Welles (with Rita Hayworth)

This year's most popular films included *A View to Kill*, a James Bond adventure with the last appearance of Roger Moore as Bond. Other hits were:

Back to The Future	Michael J. Fox and Christopher Lloyd
Witness	Harrison Ford
Pale Rider	Clint Eastwood
My Beautiful Launderette	Daniel Day Lewis and Saeed Jaffrey
The Color Purple	Danny Glover, Whoopi Goldberg and Oprah Winfrey
Out of Africa	Meryl Streep and Robert Redford

In literature, the Hull poet Philip Larkin died. He was perhaps best known for his work *The Whitsun Weddings*.

Books published this year included *Oranges Are Not the Only Fruit* by Jeanette Winterson, *Love in the Time of Cholera* by Gabriel Garcia Marquez, *The Handmaid's Tale* by Margaret Atwood, *The Cider House Rules* by John Irving and Patrick Suskind's *Perfume: The Story of a Murderer*.

Sport

In March this year rioting broke out at the FA Cup quarter-final between Luton and Millwall as hooligans tore seats from the stands and invaded the pitch. Manchester United won the FA Cup for the sixth time as they beat Everton 1–0. Kevin Moran got the first ever red card in an FA Cup Final for a tackle but cameras later revealed that he had gone for the ball and not the man. The Scotland manager Jock Stein died of a heart attack after his team's game against Wales. There was better news for England as they qualified for next year's World Cup in Mexico. In boxing, Irishman

R Routledge
Taylor & Francis Group

Barry McGuigan won the WBA Featherweight Boxing Championship, beating the Panamanian Eusabio Pedroza, and in tennis Boris Becker became the youngest-ever men's singles champion at Wimbledon at the age of 17.

Do you remember?

Spitting Image! A hugely popular satirical puppet show which debuted in 1984 and continued well into the 1990s. It won many awards for its skilful puppetry and political satire. The Prime Minister Margaret Thatcher and the Royal Family were all targets for the latex puppets. Mrs Thatcher was portrayed as a tyrant, bullying the Cabinet, and the Queen Mother was usually portrayed clutching a bottle of gin. Norman Tebbit was a leather-clad biker, Roy Hattersley was portrayed spitting profusely with every word he said and President Reagan was a nuclear-obsessed buffoon. What other characters can you remember?

Routledge
Taylor & Francis Group

1985 Personal and local events

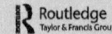
Routledge
Taylor & Francis Group

1986

Major events

January

The UK and France announced plans to build the Channel Tunnel.

Tragedy struck the US space programme when the space shuttle *Challenger* exploded and burst into flames just after take-off from Cape Canaveral. All seven astronauts died, including a female school teacher who had won a competition to be the first ordinary citizen in space.

February

Pickets clashed with police outside Rupert Murdoch's News International plant in Wapping as 5,000 print jobs were lost. Murdoch had summarily dismissed thousands of staff who went on strike at the end of January. This was to be another bitter dispute, following on the heels of the 1984/85 miners' strike and, along with legislation brought in by Mrs Thatcher, heralded the end of the power of the unions.

March

A new newspaper was launched, called *Today*. It was a tabloid to rival the *Daily Mail* and *Daily Express* and was printed in colour, which every other paper was eventually forced to adopt.

The Palace announced the engagement of Prince Andrew to Sarah Ferguson.

Catamaran services were introduced between Portsmouth and the Isle of Wight.

A fire damaged Hampton Court Palace.

April

A bill to let shops open on Sunday was defeated in the House of Commons. Many MPs felt it would damage workers' rights and have a negative impact on family life and the Church.

John McCarthy, a journalist, was kidnapped in Beirut.

The Chernobyl nuclear reactor near Kiev in the Ukraine caught fire and exploded. The leaking radioactivity contaminated a large area of Europe. The reactor was sealed in concrete.

May
Half a million black workers went on strike in South Africa.

June
The leader of Liverpool Council, Derek Hatton, was expelled from the Labour Party for membership of the Militant Tendency.

July
Prince Andrew married Sarah Ferguson (Fergie) at Westminster Abbey.

Estate agent Suzy Lamplugh disappeared.

August
Clashes between Manchester United and West Ham fans on a ferry saw English clubs banned from European competitions for another year following their ban last year after the Heysel Stadium disaster.

The National Bus Company was privatised.

One of the greatest modern sculptors, Henry Moore, died aged 88. He was known for his large smooth 'organic' forms, which were often on the theme of mother and child and executed in bronze and cement.

September
The first Japanese car plant in the UK was opened in Sunderland for Nissan cars.

October
The first edition of the *Independent* newspaper went on sale.

The Queen visited China with the Duke of Edinburgh, becoming the first British monarch to do so. Stealing the headlines, the Duke unwittingly made some inappropriate comments about Chinese eyes.

Newcastle's Metro shopping centre had its official opening, becoming the largest in Europe.

The M25 was officially opened by Mrs Thatcher.

Routledge
Taylor & Francis Group

November

Ian Brady and Myra Hindley admitted to two more moors murders.

The government launched a campaign to raise awareness of AIDS. The campaign slogan was 'Don't die of ignorance' and it angered the Church, which felt the adverts condoned sexual promiscuity.

December

British Gas shares went on sale with four million rushing to buy.

Surgeons at Papworth Hospital performed the first triple transplant (heart, lung and liver).

Also this year … scientists warned of the impending worsening of the 'greenhouse effect'. Comic Relief started this year, introducing Red Nose Day. This was also the year that the BBC's Children in Need appeal adopted Pudsey Bear as its symbol. A report this year also showed that around 10 per cent of British children were now born out of wedlock.

On the home front

With television cookery programmes doing well, more of us were willing to try 'foreign' dishes and pasta was very popular. Spaghetti Bolognese was a dinner party favourite, washed down with a bottle of supermarket Beaujolais. In the mid-1980s cheesecake would have been a very popular choice for a dinner party dessert. For the party, the fashionable hostess would probably be wearing a Zandra Rhodes design or something from Laura Ashley … labels were important! For a less formal occasion Calvin Klein jeans might be worn, as modelled by the 1980s young film star Brooke Shields of *Blue Lagoon* fame.

One of the biggest-selling books of this era was *The F-Plan Diet*, indicating that many were becoming conscious of their weight and looking to become healthier. The F stood for fibre, the idea being that you fill up on low-fat, low-calorie, high-fibre fruit, veg, pasta and potatoes. The diet industry and health concerns also saw the development of a range of low-fat products such as margarine. For the children, the sweets of the era included such delights as Cherry Lips, Fizzy Cola Bottles, Wispa bars, Caramac, Drumstick lollies and Space Dust.

Music

The most innovative album this year was Paul Simon's *Graceland*. It was recorded by Simon in South Africa with a team of black South African musicians at a time when apartheid was still a big issue. This brought some criticism, but it was lauded by others as showcasing black musicianship. It went on to become hugely successful, winning two Grammy awards with its fusion of African and Western musical styles.

Top singles this year included:

Don't Leave Me This Way	The Communards
Chain Reaction	Diana Ross
Lady in Red	Chris De Burgh
Take My Breath Away	Berlin
Walk Like an Egyptian	The Bangles
Sledgehammer	Peter Gabriel
Holding Back the Years	Simply Red
You Can Call Me Al	Paul Simon
Living on a Prayer	Bon Jovi
Walk of Life	Dire Straits
Don't Stand So Close To Me	The Police

Television

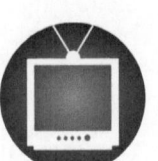

The biggest ever UK television audience of over 30 million tuned in on Christmas Day to see Dirty Den (Leslie Grantham) serve divorce papers on Angie (Anita Dobson) at the Queen Vic in *EastEnders*.

Television debuts included *Casualty*, *Bread*, the children's programme *Pingu* and *Lovejoy*. *Lovejoy* was a comedy drama with Ian McShane portraying a lovable rogue of an antiques dealer. This year also saw two remarkable drama series aired. *The Monocled Mutineer* starred Paul McGann playing soldier Percy Topliss, who went AWOL and

Routledge
Taylor & Francis Group

became a deserter. The story was based on real mutinies which occurred in 1917 at Etaples. The screenplay was written by Alan Bleasdale, who had also given us *Boys from the Blackstuff*.

The Singing Detective was another masterpiece of drama from Dennis Potter. It starred Michael Gambon as Philip Marlow, who was hospitalised due to a skin and joint disease. The story revolved around a fantasy about a novel he was creating that featured a detective called Marlow. It also encompassed his life on the ward and flashbacks to his childhood in World War II.

Screen and page

On 30 March actor James Cagney died aged 86. He made his name playing tough guy roles in films such as *Public Enemy*, *Angels with Dirty Faces* and *White Heat*.

Cary Grant died on 30 November. This English actor, born in 1904 in Bristol, went on to make it big in Hollywood. With his good looks he became a sought-after leading man and went on to make over 70 films. See how many of his films you can recall – they included *Notorious*, *To Catch a Thief*, *Charade* and *North by Northwest*.

This year's blockbuster movie was *Transformers*, which spawned many toys, but other favourite film releases included:

Top Gun	Tom Cruise
Alien	Sigourney Weaver
Platoon	Charlie Sheen
Blue Velvet	Isabella Rossellini and Denis Hopper
Crocodile Dundee	Paul Hogan
The Mission	Robert De Niro and Jeremy Irons
Labyrinth	Jennifer Connelly
Mona Lisa	Bob Hoskins

In the world of literature, Simone de Beauvoir died aged 78. She was a French feminist writer and philosopher, long-time associate of Jean-Paul Sartre and author of *The Second Sex*, a hugely respected work of feminist philosophy.

Routledge
Taylor & Francis Group

131

Books published this year included *The Old Devils* by Kingsley Amis, *A Perfect Spy* by John Le Carré, *Redwall* by Brian Jaques, *The Bourne Supremacy* by Robert Ludlum, *Batman:The Dark Knight Returns* by Frank Miller and P. D. James's *A Taste for Death*.

Sport

Argentina's Maradona 'handballed' England out of the football World Cup in the quarter-finals. Argentina went on to win, beating West Germany 3–2, but Gary Lineker won the 'Golden Boot' as the highest scorer. Lineker went on to be the most expensive British player after a transfer to Barcelona for £2.75 million. This record only lasted for a day as Ian Rush was transferred to Juventus the next day for £3.2 million. This year saw the first FA Cup Final to be a Merseyside derby. Liverpool won 3–1 after having already won the League title. Ron Atkinson was sacked and Alex Ferguson became the Manchester United manager, picking them up at second from the bottom of the First Division. In boxing, Mike Tyson became the youngest world heavyweight champion at just over 20 years old and, in golf, Jack Nicklaus won the 50th US Masters at the age of 46, beating a strong field of younger Europeans.

Do you remember?

Toys of the 1980s! Hungry Hippos was a popular game. You hit the hippo and its head extended and grabbed marbles! Lego began to appeal to the older child in 1984 with the introduction Lego Technic. This had many complicated small pieces and fiddly bits with moving parts such as cars with gears, axles and steering. One big craze was for Cabbage Patch dolls. These ugly but still cute, plump dolls were extremely popular and parents were fighting over them in the shops at Christmas 1983. The card game Top Trumps is still selling well today. Here you had themed packs of cards with facts and data about the cards' subject. You would choose a fact on your card which you thought would 'top' your opponents' cards' score. Card categories included dinosaurs, racing cars, planes, cartoon characters, etc. Probably the best game of the decade was Trivial Pursuit. It was a board game where you had to collect a set of coloured wedges by answering several categories of question such as geography, entertainment, history, literature, science and sport. In the late 1980s Teenage Mutant Ninja Turtles were popular as a comic series and cartoon, but they soon spawned a whole series of turtle-themed toys and electronic games. Other popular toys included Paul Daniels Magic Sets, Smurfs, Care Bears, Micro Machines and Jenga.

1986 Personal and local events

Routledge
Taylor & Francis Group

1987

Major events

January

Golliwogs were banned from Enid Blyton books having been deemed racially offensive.

The Archbishop of Canterbury's envoy Terry Waite was kidnapped while trying to negotiate the release of Western hostages in Beirut.

After workers going for a year without pay, demonstrations at Rupert Murdoch's News International plant in Wapping came to an end as the strike collapsed.

February

Pop artist Andy Warhol died. His famous images included colourful screen prints of Marilyn Monroe and a Campbell's soup tin.

March

Roll-on roll-off ferry *Herald of Free Enterprise* capsized off Zeebrugge, killing 188. The bow doors had not shut properly, letting water into the car deck, which made the ship keel over just outside the harbour wall.

A sale at Christie's auction rooms in London saw Van Gogh's *Sunflowers* sell for £24,750,000. This was a world record, but it fell on 11 November when another Van Gogh, *Irises*, sold for £30 million in New York.

May

A whites-only general election saw P.W. Botha and the ruling National Party retain power in apartheid South Africa.

The Iran–Iraq War intensified as a US frigate was hit by Exocet missiles.

June

The Conservative Party won the general election with a large majority, seeing Margaret Thatcher become the first British PM to be re-elected for a third term for 160 years. Roy Jenkins and Enoch Powell lost their seats while Jim Callaghan retired.

Race riots broke out in the Chapeltown area of Leeds.

Routledge
Taylor & Francis Group

July

The Docklands Light Railway was opened by the Queen. It was the first railway in the UK without drivers.

August

The SDP merged with the Liberal Party.

Ex-Nazi leader Rudolf Hess committed suicide in Spandau Prison after spending 40 years there. The prison was almost immediately demolished.

Britain's worst ever shooting occurred at Hungerford when a gunman, Michael Ryan, ran amok before shooting himself; 16 others died.

September

Severe floods in Bangladesh left 20 million homeless or facing starvation.

October

The Swedish store Ikea opened its first UK branch.

An attempt to find the Loch Ness monster using modern scanning techniques drew a blank.

Storms in south-east England with 93mph winds left many trees felled and 22 people dead.

Stock markets collapsed on what became known as 'Black Monday'. The fall in the New York stock exchange was twice that of the Wall Street crash of 1929.

November

Eleven died and many were injured when an IRA bomb exploded at a Remembrance Day service in Enniskillen.

A fire at Kings Cross underground at the end of the evening rush hour killed 30 as smoke poured through the tunnels. There was no sprinkler system in operation.

December

Presidents Reagan and Gorbachev signed an arms treaty.

Work started on the Channel Tunnel.

Also this year … unemployment was beginning to fall and a criminal was convicted on the basis of genetic fingerprinting for the first time.

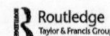

On the home front

The British-built Peugeot 405 was voted European Car of the Year, but every young pedestrian wanted to have some NIKE Air Max shoes, the first with a 'technical' sole, though I am sure those who wore the ever-popular Dr Marten boots with their air-cushioned soles would disagree. Fuelling our cars, petrol was around £1.70 a gallon, that's around 38p a litre. Fuelling our stomachs was becoming more expensive too, but cooking was a popular hobby for many. Keith Floyd had a proliferation of television cookery shows such as *Floyd on Fish* and *Floyd on France*. The 1980s could be called the era of pasta as Italian foods became very popular both to cook and when eating out! But polls indicated that chicken had replaced the roast beef joint as the nation's favourite Sunday lunch. Tastes were clearly broadening and there were more fast food outlets from various countries, more home delivery and more frozen, microwaved and ready meals available in supermarkets. In the early 1980s Sainsbury's had an average of around 7,000 products on the shelves but by the early 1990s this had risen to over 17,000. More natural fruit juices were being drunk and carbonated water was becoming very popular. Coffee was almost overtaking tea as the daily breakfast and mid-morning work break drink. Low-calorie fizzy drinks and low-alcohol beers were also coming on to the market. Some favourites from the 1980s included Wall's Viennetta, microwave popcorn, coloured pasta, pizza and Pot Noodles.

Music

'House' music was beginning to enter the mainstream. It is essentially electronic dance music with a strong, dominant repetitive beat. The Pet Shop Boys' synthesised sound was growing in popularity and they had two hits this year with *It's a Sin* and *Always On My Mind*, their version of an Elvis classic which became this year's Christmas number one.

Classic albums released this year included *The Joshua Tree* from U2, *Bad* by Michael Jackson and *Faith* from George Michael. The year's best singles included:

Never Going To Give You Up	Rick Astley
When a Man Loves a Woman	Percy Sledge
Got My Mind Set On You	George Harrison

Routledge
Taylor & Francis Group

I Wanna Dance With Somebody (Who Loves Me)	Whitney Houston
Nothing's Gonna Stop Us Now	Starship
You Win Again	The Bee Gees
Fairytale of New York	The Pogues and Kirsty MacColl
Reet Petite	Jackie Wilson
La Bamba	Los Lobos
China In Your Hand	T'Pau

The world of classical music suffered a huge loss when British cellist Jacqueline du Pré died on 19 October. Her most famous work was Elgar's Cello Concerto in E Minor.

Television

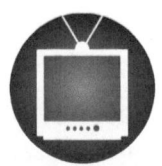

Christmas Day again got record audiences as 26 million tuned in to see Hilda Ogden's last appearance on '*Corrie*'. Jean Alexander had played the part for 23 years.

Television debuts this year included *Fireman Sam*, *The Ruth Rendell Mysteries*, *French and Saunders* and the very popular *Inspector Morse.* Morse was played by John Thaw and was a Jaguar-driving, real ale-loving, grumpy but likeable Oxford detective. His sidekick Lewis was played by Kevin Whately. On a lighter note, this year gave us *The Dame Edna Experience.*

Screen and page

This year's best film releases included *The Living Daylights* with Timothy Dalton as James Bond and the British cult film *Withnail and I* starring Paul McGann, Richard E. Grant and Richard Griffiths. Others were:

The Princess Bride	Cary Elwes
Dirty Dancing	Patrick Swayze
RoboCop	Peter Weller

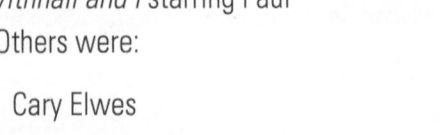

Full Metal Jacket	Matthew Modine
Empire of the Sun	Christian Bale
Wall Street	Charlie Sheen and Michael Douglas
Lethal Weapon	Mel Gibson and Danny Glover
Fatal Attraction	Michael Douglas and Glenn Close
Ironweed	Jack Nicholson and Meryl Streep
Good Morning Vietnam	Robin Williams

Several stars of the stage and screen died this year too. US actress Rita Hayworth died in May and in June the actor and dancer Fred Astaire died. Can you recall their memorable films? A third death was that of Danny Kaye. He was one of America's best-loved entertainers who was also very popular in the UK, making frequent appearances at the London Palladium. His films included *The Kid from Brooklyn*, *The Secret Life of Walter Mitty*, *White Christmas* and *The Court Jester*.

In literature, the year's best books included *The Bonfire of Vanities* by Tom Wolfe, *A Brief History of Time* by Stephen Hawking, *Hatchet* by Gary Paulsen and *The Black Dahlia* by James Ellroy.

Sport

The New Zealand All Blacks won the first Rugby Union World Cup by giving Wales their worst-ever defeat, 49–6. In boxing, 'Iron' Mike Tyson added the WBA heavyweight title to his WBC one to become the undisputed heavyweight champion of the world. Ireland's Stephen Roche won this year's Tour de France, the Tour of Italy and the Tour de Romandie, a gruelling Swiss race. Coventry City won the FA Cup for the first time with a 3–2 win over Spurs and, on a sour note, jockey Lester Piggott was jailed for three years for tax evasion.

Do you remember?

Technology. The first mobile phone came in 1983 and was a Motorola Dyna. People remember it as the huge thing used by Michael Douglas playing unscrupulous businessman Gordon Gecko in the film *Wall Street*. The phone could barely fit into his hand and certainly wouldn't fit into his pocket or briefcase! Early technology seems hugely advanced at the time it is introduced but it is surprising how fast the world of technology moves and how quickly things become dated and obsolete. Ordinary phones were evolving too, with finger dials fast disappearing to be replaced by press buttons. Cordless phones were also becoming popular, allowing you to walk from room to room as you talked!

The first Amstrad home computers came in this year too, and who would have guessed that they would be an essential feature of every household in just a few years' time as the world of mass communication and technology moved on? In the 1980s they were still used mainly for gaming, keeping personal records, compiling household lists and recording your finances. Apple Macintosh personal computers were also new on the scene, having been introduced in 1984. They improved year on year so that the one you only recently bought was soon outdated. They used 'floppy disks' for storage and transferring information between computers. These were the main method for the next two decades until they were superseded by CDs, CD-ROMs and USBs. Few youngsters today will know what a floppy disk was!

Routledge
Taylor & Francis Group

1987 Personal and local events

Routledge
Taylor & Francis Group

1988

Major events

January
Margaret Thatcher became the longest-serving British Prime Minister this century.

Australia celebrated its Bicentenary with celebrations and fireworks in Sydney harbour with the Prince and Princess of Wales in attendance. There was also a replica of the fleet which brought the first convicts 200 years ago. Two thousand local Aborigines used the occasion to protest against their poor living conditions.

February
Almost unheard of … nurses took part in a day of industrial action for better pay and more cash for the NHS. They were to win a 15 per cent pay rise in April.

Ferry workers decided to strike, bringing many ports to a standstill.

The first BBC Red Nose Day raised £15 million for charity.

May
Soviet troops began withdrawal from Afghanistan.

Dog licences were abolished.

June
US President Ronald Reagan visited the UK.

July
A gas explosion on the British oil rig Piper Alpha killed 166 people. Located 120 miles north of Aberdeen, the rescue operation was hampered by the extreme heat which could be felt up to a mile away. Most of those who died were asleep at the time and the 62 who survived did so by jumping into the sea.

The stars came out to play a concert for Nelson Mandela's 70th birthday as there were worldwide demands for his release.

Paddy Ashdown became leader of the Liberal Democratic Party, a merger of the Liberal and Social Democratic Parties.

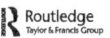

August

Iran and Iraq agreed a ceasefire.

Pubs celebrated as a new law allowed them to stay open all day.

Around 25 million were left homeless and hundreds died from more flooding in Bangladesh.

November

The US Stealth bomber, capable of being invisible to radar, made its first appearance.

December

Thirty-six died and many more were injured when two trains collided during the morning rush hour at Clapham Junction in London. An express train ran into the back of a commuter train.

Edwina Currie resigned as Health Minister after causing a scare by suggesting that most eggs were infected with salmonella.

A Pan Am Boeing 747 crashed at the small town of Lockerbie, Scotland, killing all 270 on board and 11 on the ground. The impact left a huge crater and demolished 40 houses. A terrorist bomb was found to be responsible.

Also this year ... Aids was the focus of world conferences which called for urgent action to halt the spread and find a cure. Greenpeace and other environmental groups stepped up campaigns to save whales from commercial whaling exploitation. GCSEs replaced 'O' levels. 100,000 died in an earthquake in Armenia at the end of the year, while at home the IRA continued their campaign of bombing.

On the home front

A house price boom was under way with dramatic increases in value: in some areas prices rose by over 50 per cent over the previous year. *Hello* magazine was launched, tapping into the public's fascination with celebrity. The soap opera *Neighbours* was at the height of its popularity and this was the year that one of its stars, Kylie Minogue, broke on to the pop scene. Fashion too was trying to move on by the late 1980s and more casual wear was resurfacing with the likes of sweatshirts, tracksuits and baseball boots. There were also certain subcultures which had firmly

Routledge
Taylor & Francis Group

established their own styles of fashion and looks. These were often based on musical genres and included Punk, Heavy Metal, Hip Hop and Rockabilly, and the burgeoning club scene gave clubbers the chance to experiment with lavish and bizarre styles fuelled by some of the fashion icons of the decade, such as Vivienne Westwood, Katharine Hamnett and John Galliano. Cultural magazines such as *The Face* and *i-D* were popular and helped these extravagant styles spread. Remember ra-ra skirts and parachute pants? These balloon-like eastern-style trousers were popularised by rappers and breakdancers. Stonewashed jeans were all the rage too and one of the most successful commercials from 1985 was of a young chap casually taking off his Levis and putting them into the machine at the launderette, then sitting down in his boxers to read his paper, all to the amusement of the two giggling teenage girls and other customers. Elsewhere the pint (beer) was just about to break the £1 barrier and electronic games such as Super Mario 3 were selling by the million. In the toy world, the year's must-haves were *Ghostbusters*-themed items such as slime guns!

Music

This year belonged to Bros and Kylie Minogue. Kylie was well known for her role as Charlene in the Australian soap opera *Neighbours*, so at the age of 19 she went to number one for five weeks with *I Should Be So Lucky* and had three other hits, reaching number two in the charts. Bros were a British 'boy band' who had five top ten hits this year, including a number one with *I Owe You Nothing.* Cliff Richard won the race for Christmas number one with the year's best-selling single, *Mistletoe and Wine.*

There were many other good songs around, including:

The Only Way Is Up	Yazz
He Ain't Heavy, He's My Brother	The Hollies
Heaven Is A Place On Earth	Belinda Carlisle
Orinoco Flow	Enya
A Groovy Kind Of Love	Phil Collins
Perfect	Fairground Attraction
Desire	U2

Routledge
Taylor & Francis Group

Sadly, this year on 6 December Roy Orbison died. He had a unique vocal style which was instantly recognisable and used to perform wearing trademark dark glasses. How many of these hits can you recall? His songs included *It's Over*, *Pretty Woman*, *Only The Lonely*, *Crying*, *Blue Bayou*, *In Dreams*, *Love Hurts*, *Handle with Care* and *You Got It*.

Television

Television debuts this year included *Red Dwarf*, *London's Burning*, *Wheel of Fortune* and *This Morning*. *This Morning* was a daytime television morning show which focused on 'lifestyle' issues and some current affairs. It was originally presented by Richard Madeley and Judy Finnegan.

Screen and page

Can you remember who starred in this year's best film releases?

Who Framed Roger Rabbit?	Bob Hoskins and Jessica Rabbit
Die Hard	Bruce Willis
Rain Man	Dustin Hoffman and Tom Cruise
Big	Tom Hanks
Dangerous Liaisons	Glenn Close and John Malkovich
A Fish Called Wanda	John Cleese
Dirty Rotten Scoundrels	Steve Martin and Michael Caine
Young Guns	Emilio Estevez and Kiefer Sutherland
The Last Temptation of Christ	William Dafoe

In January UK actor Trevor Howard died. He is perhaps best remembered for his role opposite Celia Johnson in *Brief Encounter*. In a prolific career, he made over 90 films. How many can you recall? They included *The Third Man*, *Mutiny on the Bounty*, *Von Ryan's Express*, *The Heart of the Matter*, *The Battle of Britain* and *Ryan's Daughter*.

The English comic actor Kenneth Williams also died this year. He is perhaps best known for his contributions to the *Carry On* series of films. His nasal tone made him quite

Routledge
Taylor & Francis Group

distinctive, especially when he uttered such phrases as, 'Ooh-er, Matron'! How many other *Carry On* cast members can you recall?

The most controversial publication this year was Salman Rushdie's *The Satanic Verses*. The book was banned in India and saw a death threat or *fatwa* against Rushdie issued by Ayatollah Khomeini of Iran. The book is a fable of good and evil but some took offence at its commentary on the prophet Muhammad. Other books published this year were *Oscar and Lucinda* by Peter Carey, *Foucault's Pendulum* by Umberto Eco, *Matilda* by Roald Dahl and *The Alchemist* by Paulo Coelho.

Sport

Florence Griffith-Joyner (Flo-jo) won the 100 metres at the Seoul Olympics. She was equally famous for running with incredibly long painted nails. The games were marred by scandal with the discovery that Canadian sprinter Ben Johnson had been taking drugs and he was subsequently stripped of his 100 metres gold medal. Great Britain and Northern Ireland won five gold medals, including Adrian Moorhouse for the 100 metres breaststroke.

Graeme Hick made cricket history by hitting 405 runs in a county match. Later the England cricket team cancelled its tour of India as many players were refused entry for taking part in a tour in apartheid South Africa.

In the Winter World Cup ski jumping competition in Canada, Great Britain's Eddie 'The Eagle' Edwards (a plasterer from Cheltenham) stole the show! He came last in both his events, finishing way behind the others, but still broke the British record in the process.

This year also saw Sandy Lyle become the first Brit to win the US Masters. And in football, after only 11 seasons in the Football League Wimbledon beat Liverpool 1–0 in the FA Cup. Elsewhere 21-year-old Paul Gascoigne transferred to Spurs from Newcastle for £2 million, a record for a British player. This was soon surpassed when Liverpool paid Juventus £2.7 million for Ian Rush, who they had sold to Juventus two years previously for £3.2 million! England crashed out of the European Championships in Germany with defeats by Ireland, the Netherlands and the Soviet Union.

Do you remember?

The late 1980s was the age of the videotape, with VHS and Betamax systems in competition with each other. Video recorders became must-haves for the home. You could also now get a camcorder to record home movies and annoy people at parties. These you could then play back via the VHS and watch/cringe together on the television. There also sprang up a proliferation of video hire shops, giving people the ability to see a wide choice of films at home. In fact, to a degree 'staying in with a video' was the new 'night out'! What videos also allowed people to do was to record their favourite television shows and soon people were building up home libraries of such recordings.

Routledge
Taylor & Francis Group

1988 Personal and local events

Routledge
Taylor & Francis Group

1989

Major events

January

Hirohito, Emperor of Japan since 1926, died aged 82.

A Boeing 737 crashed on a motorway in Leicestershire just seconds away from the runway with the loss of 44 lives.

Muslims demonstrated against the book *The Satanic Verses* by Salman Rushdie, burning the book in the streets.

George Bush (senior) was inaugurated as the 41st US President.

Spanish surrealist painter Salvador Dali died.

February

Ayatollah Khomeini issued a *fatwa* ordering Muslims to kill Salman Rushdie.

March

The oil tanker *Exxon Valdez* ruptured its tanks on reefs off Alaska, spilling 11 million gallons of oil. The ship's captain was found to be drunk at the time of the accident.

April

Ninety-five Liverpool football fans died in a crush at Hillsborough Stadium in Sheffield during an FA Cup semi-final. Too many fans were allowed into an enclosed area, causing a huge crush. The disaster led to all-seater stadiums and the end of standing on the terraces.

Chinese students held protests in Beijing demanding greater democratic freedom. A crowd of 10,000 gathered in Tiananmen Square.

Rolling Stone Bill Wyman announced he was to marry 19-year-old Mandy Smith.

May

Margaret Thatcher had been Prime Minister for 10 years.

June

Student revolt in China was brutally crushed in Tiananmen Square with tanks and public executions of demonstrators. Soldiers fired into the crowds and more than 2,000 are thought to have been massacred.

In the UK, bus, tube and rail workers went on strike.

July

The Labour Party was gaining in the opinion polls and unemployment was falling, as were house prices, but fears of a coming recession were building.

The UK experienced its hottest summer since 1976.

August

P. W. Botha resigned as South African President and was replaced by F. W. de Klerk.

Electronic tagging to monitor criminals was first used.

Fifty-one people died when the pleasure cruiser *Marchioness* collided with a dredger, *Bowbelle*, on the Thames.

It was announced that Princess Anne and Captain Mark Phillips were to separate.

September

Ambulance drivers went on strike across the UK. The police were soon having to deal with the 999 calls.

The IRA bombing campaign continued with the bombing of the Royal Marines barracks in Deal, Kent, killing 11.

October

Stock market prices fell, adding to the fear of recession.

Sixty thousand people joined an African National Congress rally in South Africa.

November

The Army were brought in to staff the ambulances.

The Berlin Wall was torn down in parts by protestors starting a mass exodus of East Germans to West Germany. This saw the East German government step down and the Berlin Wall opened. Tens of thousands fled to the West across the border, which had been closed in 1961.

Routledge
Taylor & Francis Group

The House of Commons was televised for the first time.

December

The Cold War was officially declared over this month by Margaret Thatcher, George Bush and Mikhail Gorbachev.

Margaret Thatcher won a challenge to her leadership of the Conservative Party, but her support from within the party was dwindling.

Brutal Romanian dictator Nicolae Ceausescu was overthrown and subsequently executed with his wife on 25 December, convicted of genocide.

Also this year … unemployment continued to fall to around its lowest rate of 2 million, not a situation which was to last for long as this was the height of the boom and fears of a forthcoming recession were growing.

On the home front

This was the year Rupert Murdoch launched Sky Television, for which you needed a satellite dish fixed to your house. Few at the time thought these would catch on but it was not to be long before they became a very common sight. This new service brought you many more channels and programmes than you could get with terrestrial television. Another piece of technology out this year and set to become a hugely popular and almost universal feature of childhood was the Nintendo *Game Boy*. This portable video game was simple to use. Small game cartridges were slotted in and you could play the game anywhere, or at least until the batteries ran out, but that was part of its success – you could take it anywhere. It certainly helped to brighten up long car journeys and waiting, but must have been a nightmare for teachers. Not all toys were ultra-modern and, having evolved with the fashions, Barbie was 30 this year! Adults had their own 1980s gadgets and digital watches were booming; Casio produced one with an integrated calculator. Polaroid instant cameras were all the rage too, with the film popping out just after you'd taken the shot. Great fun at parties to capture those embarrassing moments and humiliate you on the spot!

Music

Kylie and Jason Donovan had many hits throughout the year and Madonna came back into the charts with *Like a Prayer.* There was also a charity cover version of the Gerry and the Pacemakers classic *Ferry Cross the Mersey* in aid of the Hillsborough disaster victims. In the boy band world, *Bros* gave way to *New Kids on the Block* from the US, whose single *You Got It (The Right Stuff)* went straight to number one. The year's best-selling singles included:

Blame it on the Boogie	Big Fun
Ride on Time	Black Box
Swing the Mood	Jive Bunny and the Mastermixers
Back to Life	Soul to Soul
Eternal Flame	The Bangles
Too Many Broken Hearts	Jason Donovan
Especially for You	Kylie Minogue and Jason Donovan
You Got It	Roy Orbison
If You Don't Know Me By Now	Simply Red
Another Day in Paradise	Phil Collins

The year's best albums included:

The Road to Hell	Chris Rea
…But Seriously	Phil Collins
A New Flame	Simply Red
Like a Prayer	Madonna
The Raw and the Cooked	Fine Young Cannibals

Routledge
Taylor & Francis Group

Television

Dirty Den left *EastEnders*, presumed killed, thus leaving the door open for a dramatic reappearance at some future date. Television debuts this year included *Challenge Anneka*, *Byker Grove*, *A Bit of Fry and Laurie*, *Agatha Christie's Poirot* and *A Bit of a Do*. This comedy drama set in a Yorkshire town starred David Jason and followed the fortunes of two families, one working class and one middle class. Each episode was centred around a special occasion or 'do'. This year also gave us *Mr Bean*. This was Rowan Atkinson's clever creation of a bumbling immature man and harked back to the days of silent movie comedies. Another favourite comedy starting this year was *Birds of a Feather* starring Pauline Quirke, Lesley Joseph and Linda Robson. It told of the lives of two working-class women whose husbands were in jail when they moved into an expensive area in Chigwell and met their middle-class sex-obsessed neighbour Dorien.

Screen and page

This year saw the death of Samuel Beckett, the Irish writer and playwright who won the Nobel Prize for Literature in 1969, best known for his play *Waiting for Godot*. Best-selling books this year included *The Remains of the Day* by Kazuo Ishiguro, *Like Water for Chocolate* by Laura Esquivel, *The Pillars of the Earth* by Ken Follett, *A Time to Kill* by John Grisham and *The Joy Luck Club* by Amy Tan.

Can you remember who starred in these popular film releases?

My Left Foot	Daniel Day Lewis
Indiana Jones and the Last Crusade	Harrison Ford, Sean Connery
Batman	Michael Keaton, Jack Nicholson
When Harry Met Sally	Billy Crystal, Meg Ryan
The Cook, The Thief, His Wife and Her Lover	Helen Mirren, Michael Gambon
Turner and Hooch	Tom Hanks
Dead Poets Society	Robin Williams
Licence to Kill	Timothy Dalton

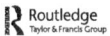

Born on the Fourth of July	Tom Cruise
Shirley Valentine	Pauline Collins and Tom Conti

This year also brought us the animated film *A Grand Day Out* with Wallace and Gromit. These characters were to become very popular over the next few years.

The actor Laurence Olivier died aged 82 this year. He was often hailed as the greatest actor of his age. His films, dating back to the 1930s, included *Wuthering Heights*, *Rebecca*, *Pride and Prejudice*, *Richard III* and *Marathon Man*.

Sport

The Hillsborough tragedy obviously overshadowed the year's sporting events but the FA Cup was allowed to run on. It was to be another Merseyside derby with Liverpool taking the spoils 3–2 and Ian Rush scoring twice. Liverpool narrowly missed taking the double as they were beaten by Arsenal with a Michael Thomas goal in the last minute of the last game of the season, giving Arsenal the League title.

In motor racing, Alain Prost won his third World Championship amid much rivalry with his team mate Ayrton Senna, who needed to win the second to last Grand Prix to get the Championship. Making a desperate attempt to overtake Prost, he ran into him five laps from the end, and went on to win but was disqualified, allowing Prost to take the Championship. Britain's Nigel Mansell won the Brazilian Grand Prix.

In boxing, Frank Bruno took on Mike Tyson for the heavyweight title of the world and lost. Englishman Nick Faldo won the US Masters, which he would also win the following year, and in the New Year's Honours list Frank Bruno and Tony Jacklin were awarded MBEs.

Do you remember?

Television advertisement slogans! A good slogan, tune or image can stick in the memory, so here is a reminder of some of the best (or worst) advertisements of the 1980s. An iconic ad for Hamlet cigars had Gregor Fisher in a photo booth frustratedly trying to brush a strand of hair over his otherwise bald head. It kept falling down as the camera flashed. Then, to the tune of Bach's *Air on a G String* he gave up, lit his cigar and disappeared under a cloud of smoke with the caption 'Happiness is a cigar called Hamlet'. Another ad which was unforgettably horrendous was for a carpet cleaner called Shake and Vac. See if you can guess the brand from the following slogans:

Vorsprung Durch Technik	*Audi cars*
I know a man who can	*Automobile Association*
Reassuringly expensive	*Stella Artois lager*
What's your favourite favourite?	*Quality Street*
… help you breathe more easily!	*Tunes*
Don't just book it …	*Thomas Cook it!*
Hello tosh, got a …	*Toshiba*
This is the age of the …	*train*
Tested by dummies	*Volvo cars*
No buts, it's got to be …	*butter*
It's a lot less bovver than a hover	*Qualcast lawnmower*
Clean kids, clean fun, clean bath	*Matey*

1989 Personal and local events

Routledge
Taylor & Francis Group

1990

Major events

January

Glasgow was this year's European Capital of Culture.

A demonstration in sympathy with the striking ambulance workers was held in London as the four-month-old strike continued.

The worst storms since 1987 battered Britain. Some 46 people were killed as hurricane force winds closed airports and ports, blew lorries over and toppled some 3 million trees.

February

Anti-apartheid campaigner Nelson Mandela was released from prison in South Africa after 27 years, at the age of 71. This followed a lifting of the ban on the African rights party, the African National Congress.

Diplomatic relations between Britain and Argentina were restored eight years after the Falklands conflict.

More storms hit, killing 14 and breaching the sea defences at Towyn, North Wales.

March

The Official Secrets Act 1989 came into force.

Violent demonstrations against the Poll Tax, which replaced the 'Rates', took place in London and elsewhere.

The ambulance strike ended after six months, with crews getting a 17.6 per cent rise.

April

A transplant doctor was struck off for using kidneys from immigrants who were paid to donate them.

Prisoners rioted at Strangeways and other prisons in protest at conditions.

May

The local elections saw Labour win more seats than the Conservatives.

After several cases of 'mad cow disease', the Agriculture Minister, John Gummer, fed his five-year-old daughter a burger on television to allay the public's fears about infected beef. France, Italy and West Germany banned British beef as a precaution.

June

The Social Democratic Party was disbanded.

July

Aldi, the German food store, opened its first UK branch in Birmingham.

An IRA bomb exploded at the Stock Exchange and later in the month a car bomb killed British MP Ian Gow.

August

Iraq invaded Kuwait, occupying the whole country and sending the ruling family into exile. The UN demanded immediate withdrawal of Iraqi troops, who had also been amassing along the Saudi Arabian border.

In the UK there was a heatwave with temperatures up to 37 degrees.

'Operation Desert Shield' saw US troops sent to the Gulf in response to a request for help from the Saudi government. Iraq held many Westerners hostage as a human shield against attack. A diplomatic solution seemed very unlikely and the UN set a withdrawal deadline of 15 January 1991.

Iraqi leader Saddam Hussein was shown on Iraq state television with British hostages, telling them they were being held to prevent war. The West saw them as being used as human shields.

Irishman Brian Keenan was released in Beirut after being held four and a half years as a hostage by Islamic kidnappers.

October

The first Wrens (Women's Royal Naval Service) to serve on an operational warship joined *HMS Brilliant*.

Routledge
Taylor & Francis Group

November

Geoffrey Howe, the Deputy Prime Minister, resigned over European policy. He later made a fierce resignation speech, attacking the Prime Minister's loathing of the EEC.

The CBI announced that Britain was in recession and Michael Heseltine said he would challenge Margaret Thatcher's leadership.

Margaret Thatcher announced that she would not fight for the Tory Party leadership and was succeeded by John Major, who beat Douglas Hurd and Michael Heseltine to the job. A tearful Mrs Thatcher left Downing Street on 28 November.

December

French and British workers shook hands 40 metres below the seabed, having dug through the Channel Tunnel.

Heavy snow brought the country to a standstill, cutting power to many in rural areas.

Lech Walesa won a landslide victory in the Polish presidential elections.

Poundland and Netto both opened their first stores in the UK.

The last coal mine in Rhondda closed after 100 years of mining in the valley. Employment opportunities for the redundant miners were few and far between.

More storms on Christmas day left many without power.

Also this year … the Hubble space telescope was launched this year from the shuttle *Discovery*. Unemployment got down to nearly 1.6 million but inflation was running at nearly 10 per cent and high street sales were at a 10-year low. The UK population was around 57 million and 10 per cent of the population was now non-white.

On the home front

A BBC survey called *Breadline Britain* found that in 1990, 93 per cent had a telephone, 82 per cent a car and 84 per cent a home computer. Yet most respondents claimed these three items were not necessities! What would be the response today? At the other end of the social scale, this was an era of supermodels and one such, Linda Evangelista, was famously quoted as saying 'I don't get out of bed for less than $10,000 a day'! Back in the real world, a Mars bar cost 20p, a pint of milk 31p

Ⓡ **Routledge**
Taylor & Francis Group

and a sliced white loaf around 46p. The average house price was £70,000 and a gallon of petrol cost around £1.86. The best-selling car was the Ford Fiesta and it was to be the most popular car of the decade. Lakeside shopping centre in Thurrock opened this year and visiting such shopping centres was a popular weekend family pastime. Many such centres had cinemas and play areas and all had many fast food outlets. The toy shops within would have been fast stocking turtles to coincide with the release of the film *Teenage Mutant Ninja Turtles.* This became a craze, spawning many a toy, and this year even one of the UK's number one singles was *Turtle Power* by Partners in Kryme!

Music

The Three Tenors, Luciano Pavarotti, Placido Domingo and Jose Carreras, gave a World Cup concert in Rome on the eve of the final. Their repertoire included the favourites *Nessun Dorma* and *O Sole Mio.* Cliff Richard had the number one spot at Christmas again with *Saviour's Day.* This made him the only person to have had a number one hit in the 1950s, 1960s, 1970s, 1980s and 1990s!

This year's other popular singles included:

Unchained Melody	The Righteous Brothers
Nothing Compares 2 U	Sinead O'Connor
Sacrifice	Elton John
Nessun Dorma	Luciano Pavarotti
The Joker	Steve Miller Band
Ice Ice Baby	Vanilla Ice
Killer	Adamski
Show Me Heaven	Maria McKee
World in Motion	New Order
A Little Time	The Beautiful South

Routledge
Taylor & Francis Group

Television

Debuts included *MasterChef*, *You've Been Framed*, *Stars in Their Eyes* and the satirical news quiz *Have I got News For You?* with Ian Hislop and Paul Merton and presented by Angus Deayton. The children's programme *Art Attack* with the very talented Neil Buchanan also debuted. Two well-loved comedies also began this year. *One Foot in the Grave* starred Richard Wilson as the grumpy Victor Meldrew, who was always finding fault with the world and others and uttering his despairing cry of 'I don't believe it!' The other comedy was *Keeping Up Appearances* with Patricia Routledge as the snobby Hyacinth Bucket, which she pronounced 'Bouquet'! This was also the year *The Simpsons* cartoon reached our screens if you had satellite television. With the lazy doughnut and beer loving Homer, who was forever uttering the curse 'Doh!' when he bungled anything, it soon became very popular. Other characters included Marge, Lisa and Bart, his naughty 'eat my shorts' son! We were also treated to another US import, *Baywatch*, which was basically some lifeguards running around with little on!

Screen and page

This year's favourite films included:

Dances with Wolves	Kevin Costner
Home Alone	Macauley Culkin
Ghost	Patrick Swayze and Demi Moore
Pretty Woman	Richard Gere and Julia Roberts
Goodfellas	Robert De Niro
Total Recall	Arnold Schwarzenegger
Edward Scissorhands	Johnny Depp
The Hunt for Red October	Sean Connery
Memphis Belle	Matthew Modine
Truly, Madly, Deeply	Alan Rickman and Juliet Stevenson

Routledge
Taylor & Francis Group

Sammy Davis Jr died this year aged 64, and also Greta Garbo, who reached the age of 84. Her career spanned the silent era and the golden age of Hollywood and her films included *Anna Karenina*, *Camille*, *Grand Hotel* and *Ninotchka*.

Popular books published this year included Nelson Mandela's *Long Walk to Freedom*, *Jurassic Park* by Michael Crichton, *Possession* by A. S. Byatt and *L. A. Confidential* by James Ellroy.

Sport

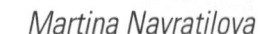

See if you can answer these 1990 sporting questions.

Which 33-year-old won a record ninth Wimbledon singles title?   *Martina Navratilova*

Who became the youngest World Snooker Champion at 21?   *Stephen Hendry*

Who won both the US Masters and the British Open?   *Nick Faldo*

At Lords, the English cricket team beat India in the highest-ever scoring Test Match. How many runs were scored?   *1,603*

Who stepped down as England manager and went out on a high, having taken England to the World Cup semi-finals? Only Alf Ramsey before him had taken England that far. They were knocked out by Germany on penalties and few will forget the sight of a tearful Stuart Pearce after his penalty miss.   *Bobby Robson*

Who did West Germany beat 1–0 in the final?   *Argentina*

Who replaced Robson?   *Graham Taylor.*

Who knocked out the previously undefeated 'invincible' Mike Tyson?   *Buster Douglas*

Who won the 100 metres in 10 seconds dead at the European Athletics Championships? Linford Christie

Routledge
Taylor & Francis Group

Do you remember?

Radio! While many have abandoned the radio for television, it remains a huge source of entertainment and news for many. The 1970s and 1980s saw a huge growth in the number of local independent radio stations, but for many the BBC stations were still the favourite ones. Radio 1 hosts the *Official Chart Show*, which started life as Alan Freeman's *Pick of the Pops* in 1967. Radio 1 show presenters of the eighties included Simon Bates and Tony Blackburn, and its popular *Breakfast Show* was fronted at times by Mike Read, Simon Mayo, Steve Wright, Chris Evans and Zoe Ball. Radio 2 is aimed at the 'older' listener and is the most listened-to station with its blend of nostalgia, news and light music. Its early morning presenters have included Jimmy Young, David Hamilton and Terry Wogan. Radio 3 is solely for classical music and Radio 4 hosts a variety of programmes, some of which have become national institutions, such as *I'm Sorry I Haven't a Clue*, *Book of the Week*, *The Archers*, *Thought for the Day*, *Desert Island Discs*, *Woman's Hour*, *Gardeners' Question Time*, *Listen with Mother*, *Test Match Special* and of course *The Shipping Forecast.*

1990 Personal and local events

Routledge
Taylor & Francis Group

1991

Major events

January

Gale force winds battered Britain, killing 27.

The Gulf War started with 'Operation Desert Storm', as US-led forces attacked Baghdad with air strikes following the passing of the deadline for an Iraqi troop withdrawal from Kuwait. The Allies launched a relentless wave of attacks that was to last a month.

Iraq paraded captured allied airmen on television.

February

An IRA mortar bomb attack on Downing Street took place but there were no injuries. Weeks later they bombed both Paddington and Victoria stations with only one death.

An allied land offensive began in Iraq and opposition collapsed. Within three days Kuwait was liberated. Saddam Hussein had set fire to all Kuwait's oil wells and all but destroyed the city.

March

The Birmingham Six, who were given life sentences for the 1974 IRA Birmingham pub bombings, were freed on appeal after 16 years in prison.

The International Olympic Committee readmitted South Africa to the Olympics after a 30-year absence.

There was a ceasefire in the Gulf, with President Bush calling for the Iraqi people to overthrow their leader Saddam Hussein. His remaining troops were still suppressing home-based rebellions of Shias and Kurds, with widespread reports of genocide.

April

The FA disclosed plans for a new 'Super' league to replace the First Division. There were fears that smaller clubs might lose out on television revenue.

May

Helen Sharman became the first Brit in space when she took part in a Russian space mission to the *Mir* space station.

Indian PM Rajiv Gandhi was assassinated.

June

War broke out in Slovenia, with battles between Serbs and Croats.

August

John McCarthy was freed in Beirut after five years as a hostage but Terry Waite was still being held captive.

September

Riots broke out in many run-down areas as unemployment reached 2.4 million. Despite this, John Major's government argued that the recession was over.

October

The courts decided that spousal rape within marriage was a crime, overturning a law that had stood since 1736 which stated that a husband could not rape his wife because she had given herself to him in the marriage contract.

November

Newspaper tycoon Robert Maxwell died in mysterious circumstances, apparently falling overboard from his yacht in the Canary Islands.

Church envoy Terry Waite was freed by Islamic extremists after four and a half years in captivity in Lebanon.

December

President Gorbachev had been temporarily deposed in Russia and Boris Yeltsin became the President of the Russian Federation. Many former republics declared themselves independent and the USSR ceased to exist.

Also this year … unemployment rose to over 2 million again with redundancies at car factories and manufacturing as the recession bit deeper. *The Times* suggested that for each vacancy there were 22 applicants. In a sign of the times, PC World opened its first

Routledge
Taylor & Francis Group

UK store. Number 1 Canada Square in Canary Wharf, with its distinctive pyramid roof and flashing aircraft warning light, became the tallest building in the UK at 770 feet or 235 metres high. The world wide web (www) was first made available to the public.

On the home front

Pizza-eating Teenage Mutant Ninja turtles were a big craze on television and film and in the toy shops. Christmas time now was not complete without a bottle of bubble bath in the shape of a Turtle character. In the world of computer games, the Mario Brothers were being rivalled by Sonic the Hedgehog! This hugely popular cult blue hedgehog ran along stinging people with his spines and jumping through hoops.

In fashion, 'puffa' jackets were popular, especially among boys to make them look bigger and tougher. They failed to see the Michelin man effect that others saw! Fashion also reflected the popularity of *Grunge*! Inspired by bands such as Nirvana, boys wore dark colours, torn jeans, army surplus, loose-fitting clothes and heavy stubble. Girls tended to wear frilly dresses with Doc Marten boots. At concerts there was much diving off the stage and crowd surfing! Older music lovers could recall strains of Neil Young and Crazy Horse. To keep fit for such activities, early risers could follow the exercise routines of Mr Motivator on GMTV. Dressed in his lurid spandex outfits and headband, the Jamaican urged viewers to join him live in his workouts. This need for exercise and weight loss became urgent as sales of the Haagen Dazs ice cream brand were boosted following sexy television ads showing semi-naked couples spoon-feeding each other!

Music

Freddie Mercury died aged 45, a high-profile victim of Aids. The subsequent re-release of *Bohemian Rhapsody* in aid of the Terrance Higgins Trust made it a huge hit for the second time. But it couldn't eclipse *(Everything I Do) I Do It For You* by Canadian Bryan Adams, which stayed at number one in the charts for 16 weeks. It was featured in the film *Robin Hood: Prince of Thieves* starring Kevin Costner. *World in Union* by Kiri Te Kanawa was commissioned by the International Rugby Football Board to represent the spirit of friendship and sportsmanship that underpins the Rugby World Cup. Other hits this year were:

The Shoop Shoop Song (It's in His Kiss)	Cher
I'm Too Sexy	Right Said Fred
Any Dream Will Do	Jason Donovan
Don't Let The Sun Go Down on Me	George Michael and Elton John
Should I Stay or Should I Go?	The Clash
Shiny Happy People	REM
Black or White	Michael Jackson

Best-selling albums this year included Chris Rea's *Auberge* and *Stars* from Simply Red.

Television

Television debuts this year included *The Brittas Empire*, *2point4 Children*, *Murder Most Horrid*, *Prime Suspect* with Helen Mirren and *Soldier Soldier*. The popular comedy drama *The Darling Buds of May* also hit the screens. This was based on the novels of H. E. Bates and centred around the exploits of the Larkin family in rural Kent. It starred David Jason as Pop Larkin, Pam Ferris as his wife (Ma) and Catherine Zeta-Jones as their eldest daughter Mariette. This year also saw Mr Blobby rise to fame in *Noel's House Party* with Noel Edmonds. This live show was set in the fictional village of Crinkley Bottom and was a mixture of funny games, children talking about their parents and CCTV secretly installed in people's homes.

Screen and page

This year's memorable films included one of the scariest for a few years. *The Silence of the Lambs*, starring Jodie Foster and Anthony Hopkins, told the story of the cannibal Hannibal Lecter and a young FBI cadet sent to interview him. He said of one of his victims, 'I ate his liver with fava beans and a nice Chianti'!

Other notable films released this year were:

The Addams Family	Anjelica Houston
Hook	Robin Williams and Dustin Hoffman

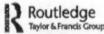

Robin Hood: Prince of Thieves	Kevin Costner and Morgan Freeman
Thelma and Louise	Susan Sarandon and Geena Davis
The Commitments	Robert Arkins
JFK	Kevin Costner

The English actress Peggy Ashcroft died this year. Her career spanned 48 years. Some will remember her from *A Passage to India* in 1984 and for winning a BAFTA that year for her role in the television series *The Jewel in the Crown*, but others will recall her as the crofter's wife in the 1935 film *The 39 Steps*.

The English novelist Graham Greene also died, on 3 April. His books included *Brighton Rock*, *The Power and the Glory*, *Our Man in Havana*, *The Third Man* and *The Quiet American*.

It was announced this year that Roald Dahl had overtaken Enid Blyton as the most popular children's author and the *Famous Five* had to give ground to *Charlie and the Chocolate Factory* and *Matilda*.

Popular books published this year included Pat Barker's *Regeneration*, *Bravo Two Zero* by Andy McNab, *American Psycho* by Brett Easton Ellis, *The Firm* by John Grisham and *Neither Here Nor There: Travels in Europe* by Bill Bryson.

Sport

In boxing, Sugar Ray Leonard, who had held five world titles, was defeated at the age of 34 by Terry Norris, 10 years his junior. After the fight he said he was going take up golf.

Manchester United won the European Cup Winners' Cup, beating Barcelona 2–1.

Liz McColgan won a gold medal at the World Athletics Championships in Tokyo for the 10,000 metres and the British men took gold in the 4×400 metres relay as Kriss Akabusi overtook the leading American down the final straight.

In the same championships, Mike Powell broke the world record for the long jump with a jump of 8.95 metres. This victory was even more significant because it broke Bob Beamon's record, which had stood for 23 years. He beat it by 5 centimetres.

The Rugby World Cup Final was won by Australia, who beat England 12–6. Many English fans felt cheated as they thought they should have had a penalty try when Australian winger David Campese deliberately knocked on. The Welsh referee only awarded a penalty and in doing so deepened the local rugby rivalry between Wales and England.

Do you remember?

Pop lyrics of the 1990s! See if you can put titles to these pop song words:

We don't talk about love, we only want to get drunk   Manic Street Preachers, 1996, *A Design for Life*

Today is gonna be the day that they're gonna throw it back to you   Oasis, 1995, *Wonder Wall*

I can eat my dinner in a fancy restaurant, but nothing, I said nothing can take away these blues   Sinead O'Connor, 1990, *Nothing Compares to You*

That's me in the corner, that's me in the spotlight   REM, 1991, *Losing My Religion*

Don't tell me it's not worth tryin' for   Bryan Adams, 1991, *(Everything I Do) I Do it for You*

I feel it in my fingers, I feel it in my toes   Wet Wet Wet, 1995, *Love is All Around*

It's coming home   The Lightning Seeds with Baddiel and Skinner, 1996, *Three Lions*

I'll tell you what I want   Spice Girls, 1996, *Wannabe*

Routledge
Taylor & Francis Group

1991 Personal and local events

Routledge
Taylor & Francis Group

1992

Major events

January
An IRA bomb exploded in Whitehall, heralding a fresh campaign that lasted all year.

Yugoslavia, formed in 1918, ceased to exist as the European Commission recognised the independence of Slovenia and Croatia. The year was to see some of the worst fighting on European soil since the Second World War as Bosnia-Hercegovina declared independence, fuelling a refugee crisis. Serb-dominated armies began a wave of 'ethnic cleansing' with the forcible mass expulsion of Bosnian Muslims. The pictures coming out reminded many of Nazi concentration camps. The Bosnian capital Sarajevo was under siege, decimating the civilian population. By the year's end and with winter fast approaching, the possibility of mass famine and a million refugees appeared likely as humanitarian aid struggled to get through.

Russian Premier Boris Yeltsin visited the UK and agreed a weapons control deal with John Major.

February
The Maastricht Treaty was signed which paved the way for the single European currency, the Euro.

March
The US sent aircraft carriers to the Gulf to pressurise Saddam Hussein into allowing the UN to inspect Iraq's nuclear facilities for weapons of mass destruction.

The Palace announced the separation of the Duke and Duchess of York.

April
The Conservatives under John Major won the UK general election, giving them a fourth term in office. Four days later Neil Kinnock announced his intention to retire as Labour leader after leading the party for over eight years.

Betty Boothroyd was elected Speaker of the House of Commons, the first woman to hold the post.

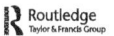

June

Baroness Thatcher took her seat in the House of Lords.

July

John Smith was elected leader of the Labour Party.

Rachel Nickell was murdered on Wimbledon Common while walking with her son. Her killer was not caught until 2008.

September

Heritage Secretary David Mellor was forced to resign following allegations of an affair.

October

The government announced the closure of more coal mines with the loss of thousands of jobs. Later in the month British Steel announced that it was to cut production due to a lack of demand.

A five-hour debate saw the General Synod of the Church of England narrowly vote in favour of the ordination of women priests. It was a debate which had divided the Church for years.

November

Bill Clinton was elected as President of the United States, ending 12 years of Republican administration.

Fire swept through Windsor Castle, destroying St George's Hall and many treasures.

December

Sixty-five people were injured in an IRA bomb attack in Manchester city centre.

The Prime Minister announced that Charles and Diana were to separate.

Also this year ... the Queen in her Christmas message described the year as an 'annus horribilis'. The Duke and Duchess of York had separated, Princess Anne had got divorced in April and Charles and Diana's marriage was on the rocks amid much media speculation and gossip. Then, to cap it all, Windsor Castle caught fire and there was an outcry when it was announced that the restoration was to be paid for out of the public purse. Elsewhere, nearly 10 per cent of the workforce were unemployed, and polytechnics became universities.

R Routledge Taylor & Francis Group

On the home front

By 1992 vinyl records were becoming a thing of the past and hard to find as CDs took over. In fashion, an advert for Calvin Klein underwear made it popular for boys to wear their jeans very low so that much of their underpants were on show! This low-slung jeans look was adopted heavily by the Rap and Hip Hop fraternity. If that isn't strange enough, Damien Hirst exhibited a pickled shark in a London art gallery, the work being entitled *The Physical Impossibility of Death in the Mind of Someone Living*. It was ridiculed by many but eventually sold for millions as an iconic example of Brit Art.

September 16 this year became known as Black Wednesday when the government withdrew the pound from the European Exchange Rate Mechanism. This cost the country billions as the pound devalued and trading losses accrued. Economic recovery was beginning as inflation was falling, though unemployment was still high and the numbers of those claiming benefits were rising fast, with some estimates putting unemployment levels at 14 per cent. Thus many families faced hard times in the early 1990s as benefit rates were well below wages and many had to apply for what was then called Supplementary Benefit to raise their 'dole' above the poverty line. Small wonder that escapism was sought by many with television programmes such as *Gladiators*, which began this year and became very popular. Contestants pitted themselves against the shows gladiators in extreme games. For those with money, new cars now came with airbags and anti-lock brakes as standard and the Ford Escort was still the best seller in the UK, followed closely by the Vauxhall Cavalier.

Music

The biggest-selling single of the year was *I Will Always Love You* by Whitney Houston, from the film *The Bodyguard* in which she starred with Kevin Costner. The soundtrack became the best-selling of all time and the song was destined to become a wedding and karaoke favourite. Other popular songs this year included:

Rhythm is a Dancer	Snap
Goodnight Girl	Wet Wet Wet

Achy Breaky Heart	Billy Ray Cyrus
Barcelona	Freddie Mercury and Montserrat Caballé
Heartbeat	Nick Berry
Stay	Shakespeare's Sister
I Drove All Night	Roy Orbison
Weather With You	Crowded House

Television

Frankie Howerd died this year, a great stand-up capable of intensely funny meandering anecdotes and best remembered for *Up Pompeii* and catchphrases such as 'Ooh-er, Missus', 'Please yourselves' and 'Titter ye not'! Benny Hill also died; his comedy relied heavily on slapstick and innuendo and he was even more popular in the US. New comedy was well in evidence with *Absolutely Fabulous* and *Men Behaving Badly*. *Absolutely Fabulous* ('Ab Fab' to fans) could almost be called 'Women Behaving Badly' as neurotic Edina, played by Jennifer Saunders, and her friend Patsy, played by Joanna Lumley, lived a life of constant shopping, drinking and parties as they tried to stay young. *Men Behaving Badly* had Martin Clunes and Neil Morrissey as flatmates equally hell-bent on not growing up despite the best efforts of their girlfriends. Other popular series debuting this year included *Heartbeat* and *A Touch of Frost*.

Screen and page

The film *Reservoir Dogs* brought director Quentin Tarantino to everyone's attention. He shot it on a comparatively small budget in only five weeks. The film centres on a robbery gone wrong and the villains attempt to find out who among them is a police informant. They all have the names of colours, such as Mr Pink, and along the way much blood is spilled in this witty but disturbing thriller. Other key films this year included:

Unforgiven	Clint Eastwood, Gene Hackman, Morgan Freeman

R Routledge
Taylor & Francis Group

Batman Returns	Michael Keaton and Danny DeVito
The Last of the Mohicans	Daniel Day Lewis
Basic Instinct	Michael Douglas and Sharon Stone
The Bodyguard	Kevin Costner and Whitney Houston
A River Runs Through It	Brad Pitt
Patriot Games	Harrison Ford

In the world of books, a controversial biography of the Princess of Wales, *Diana: Her True Story* by Andrew Morton, was published. It suggested she had made several suicide attempts after finding out that Prince Charles had resumed his relationship with Camilla Parker-Bowles. For teenagers, this year also saw the first of R. L. Stine's Goosebumps books, *Welcome to Dead House.* Other popular publications were *The Crow Road* by Iain Banks, *Fever Pitch* by Nick Hornby, *The English Patient* by Michael Ondaatje, *Band of Brothers* by Stephen E. Ambrose and John Grisham's *The Pelican Brief.*

Sport

See if you can answer these 1992 sporting conundrums:

Where were the Olympics held this year?   *Barcelona*

This year's Olympics saw the first reappearance of a unified German team and South Africa rejoined the event for the first time since 1960. With the break-up of Russia and Yugoslavia, many new states such as Croatia sent their own teams for the first time. There was also a unified team composed of former Soviet republics. Their gymnast Yevgeni Sadovi was the games' most successful athlete with six golds. What were they called?   *EUN (Equipe Unifiée)*

The games saw the first Greek sportswoman, Paraskevi Patoulidou, win a gold, but what was her event?   *100 metres hurdles*

Which British male won the 100 metres in a time of 9.96 seconds?   *Linford Christie*

Which Brit won the women's 400 metres hurdles?   *Sally Gunnell*

Who won the 4,000 metres cycling individual pursuit?   *Chris Boardman*

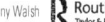

Routledge
Taylor & Francis Group

In the 400 metres semi-final a GB athlete tore a hamstring and struggled towards the finish. His father came on to the track and helped him over the line to a standing ovation. He was?   *Derek Redmond*

Who won the World Formula One Championship? He began the campaign with five straight victories and in the end won it comfortably. On his way he won the British Grand Prix at Silverstone, breaking Jackie Stewart's record of 27 wins   *Nigel Mansell*

Which pair won the Wimbledon men's and ladies' finals and went on to marry in 2001? *Andre Agassi and Steffi Graf*

In the World Snooker Championship, who beat Jimmy White 18–14?   *Steve Hendry*

Who became the UK 's most expensive footballer when he was transferred from Southampton to Blackburn Rovers for £3.6 million?   *Alan Shearer*

Do you remember?

Children's television programmes! The following list from the 1980s and 1990s should trigger a few memories.

Animaniacs, Art Attack, Blue Peter, Bob the Builder, Bodger and Badger, Byker Grove, Chucklevision, Danger Mouse, Fireman Sam, Fraggle Rock, Fun House, Grange Hill, Hey Arnold!, Live & Kicking, Power Rangers, Mike and Angelo, Pingu, Pink Panther, Postman Pat, Rainbow, Record Breakers, Roland Rat, Rosie and Jim, Rugrats, Sabrina the Teenage Witch, Scooby-Doo, Sesame Street, Teenage Mutant Hero Turtles, The Chronicles of Narnia, The Simpsons, The Smurfs, The Wide-Awake Club, Thomas the Tank Engine, Tiny Toon Adventures, Tom and Jerry, Transformers, Wizadora and ZZZAP!

Ⓡ Routledge
Taylor & Francis Group

1992 Personal and local events

Routledge
Taylor & Francis Group

1993

Major events

January
With unemployment about to exceed 3 million, the Bank of England cut interest rates to 6 per cent in an attempt to boost the economy.

Teletext replaced the Oracle.

February
Two-year-old James Bulger was abducted and murdered by two 10-year-old boys in Merseyside.

Over 1,000 died in a ferry disaster off Haiti.

March
A UN relief convoy reached Srebrenica.

The Chancellor, Norman Lamont, unveiled plans to add VAT to domestic fuel bills.

April
The Queen announced plans to open Buckingham Palace to the public.

A 51-day siege of a religious cult in Waco, Texas, ended with the death of 72 people including the cult leader and most of his followers.

Black teenager Stephen Lawrence was stabbed to death while waiting for a bus in south-east London.

An IRA bomb exploded at Bishopsgate in London, destroying a medieval church and damaging the NatWest Tower and Liverpool Street Station.

With inflation dropping, the government announced that the recession was over.

June
A high-speed train made the first run through the Channel Tunnel.

Routledge
Taylor & Francis Group

August

It was announced that for the first time the number of people on hospital waiting lists exceeded 1 million.

September

The war still raged in the Balkans, with Serbian forces besieging the Bosnian capital and later the Muslim-held town of Mostar.

The UK Independence Party was formed. It wanted to move the UK away from the European Union (as it came to be called in November this year), and the British National Party won its first council seat, in Tower Hamlets.

An Israeli–Palestinian peace accord was signed at the White House in Washington with Israeli premier Yitzhak Rabin shaking hands with PLO leader Yasser Arafat. It was supposed to give Palestinians complete autonomy on the West Bank and Gaza strip. Many were sceptical.

Also this year … inflation fell to 1.3 per cent and unemployment was finally starting to fall.

On the home front

The Ford Mondeo was the new car on the block. It was to replace the popular Sierra series. This was a large family car, a cut above the more basic Escort. It boasted a superior suspension system, luxury trim, power windows and an arm rest! It was intended to be a 'world' car and its name derived from the Latin for world, 'mundus'. It sold very well in Europe and won 1994's 'Car of the Year'. Vauxhall also launched their new Nova, which they marketed as a super-mini to replace the Corsa.

Religious practice was said to be in decline, with only one in seven people being active members of a Christian church, though many more claimed to be believers. The failure of the 'Keep Sundays Special' campaign against Sunday shopping was an indication of the general trend. There were also many other faiths with active members as immigration continued to rise, with influxes of Hindus, Sikhs and Muslims. Divorce rates were historically high and there was a rise in the popularity of cohabitation. Marriage was becoming less of an economic necessity for women as more had full-time jobs, and the number of births outside marriage was increasing. Marriage was still popular, however,

Routledge
Taylor & Francis Group

with many divorcees going on to remarry. Teenage pregnancy was seen as a growing problem and there was a rise in the number of single-parent families.

The public sector trade union UNISON was created from an amalgamation of NALGO, NUPE and COHSE. Can you remember what the initials stand for? National Association of Local Government Officers, National Union of Public Employees and Confederation of Health Service Employees. Can you remember what these other unions were? NUM, TGWU, AEEU, TUC, RMT, ASLEF, NUJ, NUT, PFA, NATFHE, NUR, USDAW and NASUWT.

In the world of fashion, Kate Moss was rising to fame as a model. She was thin, pale and waif-like, in contrast to the curvier and fuller-figured supermodels of the late 1980s and early 1990s such as Cindy Crawford and Claudia Schiffer. Away from the glamour of the catwalk, body piercings were becoming popular among certain sections of the young, with navel rings, nose studs, eyebrow and tongue piercings often being combined with tattoos.

Music

In the music world, boy bands were dominating. Take That featuring Robbie Williams and Gary Barlow had five singles in the top ten, including three number ones, all from the album *Everything Changes*. One of their hits was a song called *Relight My Fire,* which featured Lulu. The year's other best-selling singles included:

I'd Do Anything For Love	Meat Loaf
Go West	Pet Shop Boys
Everybody Hurts	REM
All That She Wants	Ace Of Base
Mr Blobby	Mr Blobby
(I Can't Help) Falling In Love With You	UB40
What is Love?	Haddaway
Dreams	Gabrielle

Television

Television debuts this year included *Breakfast with Frost* and *Peak Practice*, and the comedy game show *Shooting Stars* hosted by Vic Reeves and Bob Mortimer had its pilot episode. *GMTV* also began, presented by Eamonn Holmes. Boxing Day saw the first showing of Wallace and Gromit's *The Wrong Trousers* and was a popular Christmas feature. Christmas television has long been a mixture of old films, repeats and special programmes. Other delights of the season in 1993 included the 1942 Bing Crosby and Fred Astaire film *Holiday Inn*, *Chitty Chitty Bang Bang*, a special *Have I Got News For You?*, the inevitable *White Christmas*, *Back to the Future III* and feature-length Christmas specials of *Only Fools and Horses* and *Birds of a Feather*.

On the radio, Terry Wogan returned to Radio 2 with *Wake Up To Wogan*. It became the most listened-to breakfast show in the UK at the time.

Screen and page

The Steven Spielberg film *Jurassic Park* came out this year. With fantastic special effects bringing dinosaurs back to life, it told the story of a millionaire played by Richard Attenborough opening a theme park on an island which featured cloned dinosaurs. A storm knocks out the park's security systems and the dinosaurs go on the rampage. Other notable films were *The Crying Game*, *Unforgiven*, *Schindler's List*, *Tombstone*, *Free Willy*, *Mrs Doubtfire* and *Groundhog Day*.

The actress Audrey Hepburn died this year from cancer. As well as having a glittering Hollywood career, she was also regarded as a fashion icon. Her films included *Roman Holiday*, *Breakfast at Tiffany's*, *My Fair Lady* and *Charade*.

This year also saw the death of William Golding at 82, the author of the classic *Lord of the Flies*. The year's publications included *Bolt* by Dick Francis, Sebastian Faulks' *Birdsong*, Irvine Welsh's *Trainspotting*, *The Client* by John Grisham and *Honour Among Thieves* by Jeffrey Archer.

Routledge
Taylor & Francis Group

Sport

Three young deaths overshadowed this year's sport. James Hunt, the 1976 Formula One world champion, died of a heart attack aged just 45. He was a much-loved figure, had a liking for nightclubs and girls and led a playboy lifestyle. Arthur Ashe also died, aged 49, having tragically contracted Aids following a heart operation. Finally, one of England's best-loved footballers, the World Cup and West Ham captain Bobby Moore, died of cancer aged 51.

In football, Eric Cantona joined Manchester United from Leeds and started scoring prolifically, helping United to win the League. This victory also made Alex Ferguson the first manager to have won the League Championship in both Scotland and England. The England team failed to qualify for the 1994 World Cup in the US and manager Graham Taylor was lambasted by the press and resigned.

This year's Grand National was a fiasco because after a false start most of the runners carried on and seven completed the course. The Jockey Club decided to void the race. The jockey and owners of Esha Ness who won the race must have been somewhat aggrieved, as the horse achieved the second fastest time ever! The race was not rerun.

The Yugoslav tennis player Monica Seles was stabbed by a Steffi Graf fan at a tournament in Hamburg. She was world number one at the time but was so traumatised she struggled to consistently reproduce her best form, although she did go on to win the 1996 Australian Open.

Do you remember?

Beanie Babies! These were soft toy animals stuffed with plastic 'beans', which could be posed. They covered the whole range of animals from frogs to bears to baboons to pigs. Each had a name such as Patti the Platypus, and had heart-shaped labels attached to them. They soon became very collectible.

Polly Pocket dolls! These were small plastic hand-size cases like a tiny dolls' house with minute dolls and furniture inside.

Pogs! These were small plastic discs which came free with crisps and had cartoon characters on one side. You could play games with them but most people just tried to collect them.

Routledge
Taylor & Francis Group

1993 Personal and local events

Routledge
Taylor & Francis Group

1994

Major events

January

Forest fires were burning out of control in New South Wales, Australia, destroying over 200 homes.

The Duchess of Kent converted to Catholicism, the first royal to do so for over 300 years.

February

Seventy were killed and over 200 injured in a mortar attack in Sarajevo marketplace in the worst atrocity of the Bosnian War. This was followed throughout the month with more atrocities and NATO forces shooting down Serbian planes over Bosnia.

Police stared excavating the garden of Fred West who, it was later found, had raped, murdered and buried his daughter there. He later admitted to 10 more murders with his wife Rosemary.

April

The President of Rwanda was killed in a plane crash, triggering a bloody civil war with most violence aimed at the Tutsi minority. It went on to claim over half a million lives and create 1.5 million refugees.

Ex-president Richard Nixon died of a stroke aged 81.

Multi-racial elections began in South Africa. This essentially marked the end of 350 years of white domination of South Africa's black majority.

May

The local elections saw the Conservatives lose heavily, despite signs of economic recovery and falling unemployment.

The 31.5 mile long Channel Tunnel was opened by the Queen and President Mitterand.

Nelson Mandela was sworn in as President of South Africa after victory for his African National Congress Party.

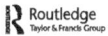

UK Labour leader John Smith died of a heart attack aged 56.

Jacqueline Kennedy Onassis died.

June
The fiftieth anniversary of the D Day landings occurred.

Norman Fowler, the Chairman of the Conservatives, resigned a few days after they performed very poorly at the European elections.

July
Tony Blair was elected leader of the Labour Party, beating competition from John Prescott and Margaret Beckett. Labour were by now way ahead in the opinion polls.

August
The IRA announced a ceasefire in Northern Ireland.

October
The 'cash for questions' scandal broke as Conservative MPs were accused of taking bribes from Harrods' owner Mohamed Al-Fayed to ask questions in the House of Commons.

November
The first National Lottery draw took place in the UK.

December
Russian aircraft bombed the Chechen capital, Grozny, in an effort to crush the independence movement.

Also this year … VAT on fuel bills was introduced.

On the home front

The Sony PlayStation was launched this year in Japan; in Europe we had to wait until 1995 for it to become available, but gamers' mouths were watering. You hooked the console up to your PC and played with the hand-held controller. It was so big an advance in gaming and so sought after that in its first 10 years it sold over 100 million. There were thousands of different games you could buy to play. It is fondly remembered as the PS1 and compared with modern versions it now seems a bit tame.

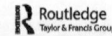

On a more personal front, bra sales rocketed after the Wonderbra ad featuring Czechoslovakian model Eva Herzigova in her underwear. This appeared on billboards around the world with the slogan 'Hello boys'! Other popular 1990s fashion items included the lycra dresses and bandeau bra dresses worn to indulge the other 1990s craze of salsa and lambada dancing. Many evening classes emerged to teach these sensual rhythmic dances. The other dance craze at this time was a US import, line dancing. Here mixed-sex rows of dancers dressed in cowboy outfits assiduously followed (or tried to follow) the master of ceremonies' instructions to create a sort of upright linear Busby Berkeley effect!

Music

Mariah Carey had four hits in the top ten this year, including *Without You*, which had been a hit for Harry Nilsson in 1971. She also had a big Christmas hit with *All I Want For Christmas Is You.* The biggest hit was *Love is All Around* by Wet Wet Wet, which spent 15 weeks at the top, helped by its use in the film *Four Weddings and a Funeral.* Another boy band, Boyzone, were beginning to emerge with a version of the Osmonds' song *Love Me For A Reason.* In the album charts, Manchester band Oasis shot straight to number one with their debut album *Definitely Maybe.* Other hits included:

Stay Another Day	East 17
Baby Come Back	Pato Banton
Always	Bon Jovi
Crocodile Shoes	Jimmy Nail
The Power of Love	Celine Dion
Cigarettes and Alcohol	Oasis

Television

Television debuts this year included *Animal Hospital* with Rolf Harris, *Ready Steady Cook* and the popular archaeology programme *Time Team* with Tony Robinson. On children's television, the excellent art programme *SMart*, presented by the talented Mark Speight, was growing in popularity, but the biggest television event of the year was the first showing of the comedy *The Vicar of Dibley.* This had Dawn French playing the newly appointed female vicar to the rural parish of Dibley. It had many memorable characters, including Alice the 'dippy' verger and Hugo, her equally dim-witted boyfriend. Two of the other parishioners were Owen, the local farmer with poor personal hygiene and an over-fondness for his animals, and Jim, a lecherous pensioner with a confusing stutter, 'n...n...no...no...no...n...yes'! In the world of investigation, *The X-Files* began this year and soon became cult viewing. FBI agents Mulder and Scully investigated cases of inexplicable phenomena or paranormal activity which were filed by the FBI under 'X'. The show's catchphrase was 'The truth is out there'.

Screen and page

Popular films this year included:

Four Weddings and a Funeral	Hugh Grant, Andie MacDowell and Simon Callow
The Shawshank Redemption	Tim Robbins and Morgan Freeman
Pulp Fiction	John Travolta, Samuel L. Jackson and Uma Thurman
Forrest Gump	Tom Hanks
The Lion King	Animation
Natural Born Killers	Woody Harrelson and Juliette Lewis
Dumb and Dumber	Jim Carrey and Jeff Daniels
The Flintstones	John Goodman

The veteran Hollywood actor Burt Lancaster died this year aged 80. He made over 75 films, including *From Here To Eternity*, *Apache*, *Vera Cruz*, *Trapeze*, *Elmer Gantry*, *The Birdman of Alcatraz* and *Local Hero*.

Routledge
Taylor & Francis Group

In the book world, this year saw the publication of *Captain Corelli's Mandolin* by Louis de Bernières, P. D. James's *Original Sin*, *A Suitable Job for a Woman* by Val McDermid and *Snow Falling on Cedars* by David Guterson. In the world of comic books, in the US the popular *Hellboy: Seed of Destruction* was published and soon became a cult phenomenon. A decade later it was to spawn several films. The book *Prozac Nation* by Elizabeth Wurtzel also became something of a phenomenon, describing the author's battle with depression.

Sport

Over two days the world of motor racing lost the Brazilian champion Ayrton Senna and Austrian driver Roland Ratzenberger in two separate crashes on the same stretch of track at the San Marino Grand Prix.

The Winter Olympics in Lillehammer were embroiled in controversy and histrionics between Nancy Kerrigan and Tonya Harding. Early in the year Kerrigan had been attacked by Harding's ex-husband in an attempt to break her leg, forcing her to withdraw from the US national championships, which Harding won, only to be later stripped of the title because of the attack. She came eighth in the Winter Olympics figure skating, but Kerrigan had the last laugh, taking the silver medal.

Following Graham Taylor's resignation the previous year, Terry Venables was appointed England football manager. In the World Cup in the US, Maradona failed a drug test and was sent home. Even worse, Columbian footballer Andres Escobar scored an own goal against the US, leaving little hope of Columbia's qualifying for the final stages. On his return home he was gunned down and killed. It is alleged that drug barons lost millions in bets as a result of his unfortunate own goal.

Coming out of retirement after 10 years, George Foreman at 45 became the oldest man to win the world heavyweight title as he knocked out Michael Moorer, 18 years his junior, who had taken the world title from Evander Holyfield. Most commentators thought the whole thing was a farce, but ended up with egg on their faces as Foreman, well behind on points, won it with only seven minutes to go.

Two losses this year were 1976 world and Olympic skating champion John Curry, who died of Aids, and the footballing legend Sir Matt Busby, who died aged 84.

 Routledge Taylor & Francis Group

Do you remember?

1990s holidays! Since about 1994 Spain and its 'Costas' have been the most popular holiday destination for Brits looking to go abroad, though by the 1990s a few more were exploring Greece and Turkey. With cheap package deals it was often cheaper than staying at home and had the added advantage of guaranteed sunshine and hot weather. Spanish holiday resorts offered a mixture of hotel accommodation, discos, cheap food and drink and of course warm sunny beaches and a warm sea. Holiday camps were in decline because of such cheap overseas attractions and even the USA was within range for some. By the mid-1990s only three Butlins camps remained and they were in need of some serious overhauls and rebranding. Ten million were taking overseas package deals in 1986 and by 2003 it would be double that. Benidorm was a typical destination. A sleepy fishing village in the 1960s, by now it was huge and full of skyscrapers and hotels, due entirely to the tourism boom in the 1970s and 1980s. Its reputation was tarnished because of British lager louts, despite the tourist companies' efforts to market packages as family holidays. Club 18–30 was also doing very well in the mid-1990s, with its emphasis on 'fun'! But for most families the package bought them a memorable Spanish experience and souvenirs of sombreros, sangria and toy bulls.

1994 Personal and local events

Routledge
Taylor & Francis Group

1995

Major events

January

Five thousand died in an earthquake in Kobe, Japan, which also left 250,000 homeless.

Cave paintings 20,000 years old were found in southern France.

The O. J. Simpson trial began in Los Angeles. Simpson was charged with the murder of his ex-wife and a male companion, but was eventually acquitted.

February

Barings Bank in London went into receivership after trader Nick Leeson lost £860 million on Japanese markets. He fled to Singapore but was subsequently jailed for six and a half years.

March

The Queen visited Northern Ireland for the first time since the ceasefire. She also visited South Africa and met Nelson Mandela.

April

British troops prepared to leave Northern Ireland.

May

Local elections saw the Conservatives left with control of only eight councils.

It was the fiftieth anniversary of VE Day.

June

John Major resigned as leader of the Conservative Party in order to test his leadership support in the face of internal criticism. He won the subsequent election by a large majority.

The US space shuttle *Atlantis* docked with the Russian space station *Mir*.

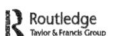

August
The fiftieth anniversary of VJ Day took place.

UN forces attacked key Serbian positions.

October
President Bill Clinton and his wife Hillary visited England, Northern Ireland and the Republic of Ireland.

November
Israeli Prime Minister Yitzhak Rabin was assassinated after addressing a peace rally. He had been a marked man for extremists from the moment he shook hands with Yasser Arafat on the steps of the White House in 1993.

The Queen Mother had a hip replacement at the age of 95.

The newspaper *Today* folded after just nine years in print.

A ceasefire was declared in Bosnia.

Kenneth Clarke, the Chancellor, cut the basic rate of income tax to 24p.

Also this year ... a link was found between BSE in cattle and CJD in humans, giving rise to the term 'mad cow disease'. The war in Chechnya carried on despite near-universal condemnation by the rest of the world, leaving Boris Yeltsin's Russian presidency with limited credibility. Despite the decimation of the capital, Grozny, the Chechen guerrillas vowed to fight on. Torrential rain brought widespread flooding to parts of northern Europe such as the Netherlands, with a quarter of a million evacuated.

On the home front

The top new car was the Vauxhall Vectra, which replaced the Cavalier. Just the thing for popping over to the Isle of Skye, whose bridge linking it to the mainland was completed this year at a cost of £25 million. Many were not in favour of the bridge, arguing that it took away some of the mystery of the island and there were realistic fears over ferry job cuts. The Vectra was not in this year's best-selling car top ten, but its predecessor was. The list is:

Routledge
Taylor & Francis Group

Ford Escort	Vauxhall Corsa
Ford Fiesta	Rover 200
Ford Mondeo	Peugeot 306
Vauxhall Astra	Renault Clio
Vauxhall Cavalier	Rover 100

Over the decade the Fiesta comes out as the best-selling car, closely followed by the Escort and Astra. The best car advert, though, must go to the Renault Clio as used by 'Papa' and 'Nicole'! These fictional characters were featured throughout the 1990s and developed their own storylines over the years. The finale in 1998 had Nicole being led down the aisle, then leaving Vic Reeves standing at the altar as she ran off with Bob Mortimer in his new Renault Clio. Screened during a break in *Coronation Street*, the ad was seen by over 20 million people.

Music

After countless hit records, Cliff Richard becomes Sir Cliff! This year the Irish boy band Boyzone had the most top ten entries with songs such as *Father and Son*, and Oasis were enjoying a wave of more Rock-oriented hits. The biggest-selling single was *Unchained Melody by* Robson and Jerome, the television stars from *Soldier Soldier.* Other top singles included:

Back for Good	Take That
Wonderwall	Oasis
It's Oh So Quiet	Björk
Don't Stop (Wiggle Wiggle)	The Outhere Brothers
Hold Me, Thrill Me, Kiss Me, Kill Me	U2
A Girl Like You	Edwyn Collins
You Are Not Alone	Michael Jackson
Fairground	Simply Red
Missing	Everything But The Girl

 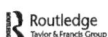 Routledge
Taylor & Francis Group

Best-selling albums included *(What's the Story) Morning Glory?* by Oasis, *Stanley Road* by Paul Weller, *The Great Escape* by Blur and Celine Dion's *The Colour of My Love*.

Television

Television debuts this year included *Can't Cook, Won't Cook,* with chef Ainsley Harriott and the funny sports quiz *They Think It's All Over* hosted by Nick Hancock and with team captains David Gower and Gary Lineker. One of the rounds was called 'Feel the Sportsman', where the captains were blindfolded and had to guess who the guest personality was! Another comedy series starting out was the popular *Father Ted*, an Irish comedy about a group of priests living together on a remote island. *Hollyoaks*, a new soap opera, also began. This was set in a suburb of Chester and focused more on younger people than other soaps. Elsewhere in 'Soapland', Julie Goodyear aka barmaid Bet Lynch left *Coronation Street* after a spell of almost 30 years. This year also gave us Wallace and Gromit in *A Close Shave,* but the television sensation of the year was a frank interview given by the Princess of Wales on the BBC's *Panorama*. She spoke candidly about adultery, her depression, bulimia and children. Nearly 30 million tuned in to watch it. Sadly, this year Peter Cook died aged 57. He was a founder of *Private Eye* and a great satirist, best known for his television partnership with Dudley Moore in *Not Only But Also.*

Screen and page

Pierce Brosnan became James Bond as the spy returned to the screen after an absence of six years in the 16th Bond film, *GoldenEye*. This year's popular releases included:

Braveheart	Mel Gibson
Se7en	Morgan Freeman and Brad Pitt
The Usual Suspects	Kevin Spacey and Gabriel Byrne
Toy Story	
Jumanji	Robin Williams and Kirsten Dunst
Apollo 13	Tom Hanks

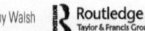

Waterworld	Kevin Costner
Casper	
The Englishman Who Went Up a Hill But Came Down a Mountain	Hugh Grant

In literature, this year's best sellers included *The Ghost Road* by Pat Barker, *Northern Lights* by Philip Pullman, Nick Hornby's *High Fidelity*, James Patterson's *Kiss the Girls* and the very funny American take on the UK, *Notes from a Small Island* by Bill Bryson.

Sport

Steffi Graf won her sixth Wimbledon ladies' title in the year that Fred Perry died. In boxing, Frank Bruno won the WBC World Heavyweight Championship, but he was to lose it next year to Mike Tyson, who stopped him in the third round. In athletics, Jonathan Edwards set a new world triple jump record (twice) and became BBC Sports Personality of the Year.

Playing in the World Cup for the first time, South Africa won the Rugby World Cup on 25 June. They beat a formidable New Zealand side which included the man of the tournament, Jonah Lomu. They were watched by 43 million on television and 60,000 at the game in Johannesburg. None was more pleased than Nelson Mandela, who presented South Africa with the Cup.

In football, Manchester United's Eric Cantona was sent off and launched a flying Kung Fu-style kick at a Crystal Palace fan who verbally abused him. He was banned for the rest of the season. There was also more crowd violence with 800 Chelsea fans being deported from Belgium, and a friendly against Ireland was abandoned because of rioting English fans. This year also saw Bruce Grobbelaar and Justin Fashanu investigated for match fixing.

In Formula One, Michael Schumacher won his second Grand Prix Championship, with his nearest rival, England's Damon Hill, in second place.

Do you remember?

Crazes of the 1990s! There were quite a few. Line dancing took off with the Billy Ray Cyrus song *Achy Breaky Heart*, whose 1992 video was a well-choreographed line dance. The video to Madonna's 1990 hit *Vogue* was a tribute to the 'vogue' dance style where dancers adopt model-like poses with rigid arm, leg and body movements! The Union Jack became a fashion icon again in the 1990s with the phrase 'cool Britannia' referring to a resurgence of British fashion and music. Exemplifying this were Geri Halliwell's Union Jack dress and bands such as Oasis with Noel Gallagher's Union Jack guitar. The Spice Girls were also responsible for the phrase 'girl power'. Another phenomenon of the 1990s was the so-called Magic Eye. These were abstract images which revealed hidden pictures if you stared at them in a certain way. Some people could do it straight away but others, try as they might, could not pick out the hidden image. Originating in the late 1980s, *Where's Wally?* was now very popular. These picture books of crowd scenes had 'Wally' in his red and white hooped shirt and walking stick hidden somewhere within. Wally had local names, so that in the US he was Waldo, in Germany he was Walter and in Czechoslovakia he was Valdik. He was later joined by a girl called Wenda and a dog called Woof, all similarly attired.

Routledge
Taylor & Francis Group

1995 Personal and local events

1996

Major events

January

The Conservatives remained in power but the polls indicated that Labour were well ahead in the public opinion stakes.

February

Genetically modified food went on sale in the UK for the first time.

The IRA ceasefire ended with a bomb under a railway station in London's docklands, throwing the Irish peace process into jeopardy. Forty were injured and two died.

A thousand passengers were trapped in the Channel Tunnel when two trains broke down. The fault was electrical problems caused by snow and ice.

March

A massacre took place in Dunblane, Stirling, when 16 children and a teacher were shot dead in the primary school gym by a deranged gunman who then shot himself. He wounded 13 other children and another teacher.

British beef was banned by Europe following the government's admission of a possible link between BSE and 'mad cow disease' or CJD, a human brain disease.

A ceasefire was achieved in Chechnya.

April

The Conservative majority in Parliament was cut to just three seats as Labour won another by-election.

May

The Conservatives lost heavily in the local elections.

The Duke and Duchess of York divorced.

June

An IRA bomb caused a huge explosion to rock the Arndale shopping area in central Manchester. Two hundred were injured, many by broken glass. The ceasefire was well and truly over. The army were trying to examine a suspect van when it exploded. John Major urged Sinn Fein to condemn the attack and demanded a ceasefire.

July

Dolly the sheep was born, the first successfully cloned mammal.

Nelson Mandela visited London.

A bomb at the Atlanta Olympics killed two and injured 111. The Atlanta Olympics, though, will best be remembered for the sight of a trembling Muhammad Ali lighting the Olympic flame. He was suffering from Parkinson's disease.

August

The Prince and Princess of Wales divorced after 15 years of marriage. Irreconcilable differences were cited as both had publicly admitted adultery.

November

Bill Clinton was re-elected as US President.

A fire in the Channel Tunnel disrupted services.

The Stone of Scone arrived back in Edinburgh Castle after it was removed by King Edward 1,700 years ago.

Also this year ... unemployment fell below 2 million and the Conservative government ended the year without a majority in the House of Commons.

On the home front

Following the success of the animated film *Toy Story*, demand for Buzz Lightyear toys at Christmas was such that supplies ran out. For those with more money to spend, Ford launched their new Ka. This was a small runaround city car nicknamed the 'egg' car. The three-door hatchback soon became very popular for city drivers. The average house price was £70,000 and a gallon of petrol cost £2.70. Mobile phones were by now commonplace and still quite large, but reception was improving.

Routledge
Taylor & Francis Group

The burden of housekeeping was still primarily the responsibility of women, but more home appliances were becoming available and were seen as liberating housewives from hours of household chores. However, the housework still needed to be done! We might have a washing machine but we all had more clothes! The increase in kitchen gadgets meant that we spent less time cooking and more time eating fast foods using microwaves and pre-prepared convenience foods. Toasters, slow cookers and blenders were necessary as more and more families became dual-income families so there was less time for cooking. Even decorating trends suggested a more minimalist, less cluttered, low-maintenance approach. There was lots of easy-to-clean stainless steel and Scandinavian-style pine furniture was popular. Kitchens were mainly white with built-in cupboards and clever storage solutions to keep things looking sparse. In the living room the 1980s had seen a penchant for dense floral wallpapers and wall-to-wall carpets, but in the 1990s wooden floors were increasingly preferred alongside the pine furniture.

Music

Teenage girls were shocked this year to find that Robbie Williams had left the boy band Take That, but were somewhat comforted as girl power came on the scene with the Spice Girls, who had three number ones this year, *Wannabe*, *Say You'll Be There* and *2 Become 1*. Can you name the Spice Girls and their alter egos? Geri Halliwell was Ginger Spice, Melanie Chisholm was Sporty Spice, Melanie Brown was Scary Spice, Emma Bunton was Baby Spice and Victoria Adams was Posh Spice.

Other hits were:

Three Lions	Baddiel and Skinner and The Lightning Seeds (the official song of the England football team)
Don't Look Back In Anger	Oasis
Killing Me Softly	The Fugees
Spaceman	Babylon Zoo
How Deep Is Your Love?	Take That
Words	Boyzone

Routledge
Taylor & Francis Group

Breathe	The Prodigy
Fast Love	George Michael

Television

Television debuts this year included *Ballykissangel, Changing Rooms, Dalziel and Pascoe* and *This Life. This Life* was a drama about the lives and loves of a group of young aspiring lawyers living in a trendy London house. It became very popular, as did the music panel game *Never Mind the Buzzcocks*, hosted by Mark Lamarr with team captains Bill Bailey and Phil Jupitus. Another debut, *TFI Friday*, was a late-night anarchic celebrity gossip and chat show hosted by Chris Evans. *The Simpsons* came to terrestrial television and *Coronation Street* went to four episodes a week. A Christmas special of *Only Fools and Horses* called *Time on Our Hands* was to be the last in the series and saw Rodney and Del Boy finally become millionaires as they sold an old watch for millions at Sothebys, much to their surprise. It was the most watched programme of the 1990s apart from the following year's funeral of Princess Diana.

Screen and page

Trainspotting, based on the novel by Irvine Welsh, starred Ewan McGregor and told the story of Edinburgh junkies in a gritty way. It also starred Robert Carlyle as the violent alcoholic Begbie. For younger viewers, the film of the year was *Toy Story* with Woody and Buzz Lightyear. Other films included:

Independence Day	Will Smith
From Dusk Till Dawn	George Clooney
Matilda	Danny DeVito
Star Trek: First Contact	Patrick Stewart
Mission: Impossible	Tom Cruise
The English Patient	Ralph Fiennes and Juliette Binoche
101 Dalmations	Glenn Close
James and the Giant Peach	

R Routledge
Taylor & Francis Group

In literature, best sellers published this year included *Angela's Ashes* by Frank McCourt, *Bridget Jones' Diary* by Helen Fielding, *Into the Wild* by John Krakauer, *The Green Mile* by Stephen King and Graham Swift's *Last Orders*.

Sport

Some 1996 sporting conundrums to solve:

The 1996 Olympics were held where?   *Atlanta, Georgia, USA*

How many gold medals did Great Britain win? And what for?   *One: Matthew Pinsent and Steve Redgrave in the men's coxless pairs*

Great Britain won three worthy silver medals for javelin, 400 metres and triple jump. Who won these?   *Steve Backley, Roger Black and Jonathan Edwards*

Who won two gold medals, for 200 and 400 metres?   *Michael Johnson*

Who won his fourth long jump gold medal at the age of 45?   *Carl Lewis*

Who won the Japanese Grand Prix in October and the Formula One World Championship, thus following in the footsteps of his father Graham?   *Damon Hill*

In boxing, who knocked out Frank Bruno in the third round to win the WBC heavyweight title?   *Mike Tyson*

Who stopped Tyson in the 11th round later that year?   *Evander Holyfield*

England hosted Euro 96 and almost inevitably lost a penalty shoot-out in the semi-finals. To whom?   *Germany*

Who did Germany go on to beat in the final?   *The Czech Republic*

The England manager resigned but the team only lost once under his leadership. He was?   *Terry Venables*

Who replaced him?   *Glenn Hoddle*

Which five times British champion Scottish jockey retired this year after a bad fall? *Willie Carson*

Routledge Taylor & Francis Group   **209**

Do you remember?

Tamagotchi? This was a popular interactive toy – basically an electronic pet which was touch, sound and light sensitive and had to be looked after. It was small enough to fit into the palm of your hand and had a display screen. On first activating it you got a picture of an egg which wobbled a bit and then hatched into your pet. You then basically had to care for it as it grew up. It needed feeding, exercising and cleaning up after like a real pet. It left droppings on the screen which you had to clean up and if you didn't do this, feed or otherwise look after it, it would get ill and even die. They did not go down well at school as at the sound of a beep children would realise they needed to get them out of their pockets and attend to their needs! The word is Japanese and means a watch in an egg!

Another popular 1990s icon was *Tomb Raider.* This was a video game and appealed to both teenage boys and girls. Tomb Raider was Lara Croft, a buxom archaeologist adventurer in hot pants with pistols strapped to each thigh! She travelled the world in search of ancient relics and had to face tasks and challenges in underground tombs, collecting items along the way. The game sold millions of copies and was turned into a film starring Angelina Jolie.

Routledge
Taylor & Francis Group

1996 Personal and local events

Routledge
Taylor & Francis Group

1997

Major events

January

The Princess of Wales began her campaign against landmines, calling for an international ban.

'Swampy' and other environmental protesters were evicted from tree houses and tunnels on the site of the new A30 by specialist climbing and caving experts. They were dubbed 'eco warriors' by the media as they used direct action to protest against road expansion.

February

Dolly the cloned sheep was presented to the world. She was cloned from a single cell of her mother. Elsewhere this month a court of appeal gave a Leeds woman the right to be inseminated with her dead husband's frozen sperm two years after his death.

March

Unemployment was down to its lowest level since 1990 at 1.8 million.

Channel 5 was launched.

May

Tony Blair's New Labour won the general election with a landslide victory. He became the youngest Prime Minister for 150 years in the largest-ever anti-government swing, giving the Labour Party their biggest-ever majority in the House of Commons. The election also put more women in Parliament than ever before.

June

William Hague was elected Tory leader, its youngest for 200 years.

Undersea explorer and inventor of the scuba diving aqualung Jacques Cousteau died.

July

Hong Kong ceased to be a colony and was officially handed over and returned to Chinese sovereignty after 99 years under British rule.

The IRA declared another ceasefire in the run-up to all-party peace talks scheduled later in the year.

August

Princess Diana was killed in a car crash aged 36, sparking a national outpouring of grief unprecedented in living memory. Her lover Dodi Fayed, son of the Harrods owner, was also killed in the car with her. It is believed the car was trying to escape the following cars full of paparazzi photographers, but their driver was also three times over the French drink-driving limit. Huge mounds of flowers and tributes were laid at the gates of royal palaces.

September

Mother Teresa of Calcutta died at the age of 87.

The funeral of Princess 'Di' took place She was described by Tony Blair as the 'people's princess'. More than 1 million lined the route and it was watched by an estimated 2 billion worldwide. Following an unprecedented week of mourning, the four-mile funeral procession brought her coffin to Westminster Abbey where the service featured Elton John singing a rewritten version of *Candle in the Wind*.

October

Thrust set a first supersonic land speed record at just over 763 mph. It was the first time the sound barrier had been broken on land.

Louise Woodward, a 19-year-old English au pair, was found guilty of the manslaughter of an eight-month-old child in her care in the USA, but freed on appeal 10 days later.

November

Brazil refused to extradite Great Train Robber Ronnie Biggs.

Also this year ... a survey showed that UK rail fares were the highest in the world. The beef crisis deepened. HMP Weare (a prison ship) was used in Portland harbour to ease congestion in prisons. The use of prison ships dates back to the 18th century when old 'hulks' were used; they could still float but were unseaworthy.

On the home front

In the 1990s the drinks market was getting some colourful new additions with the likes of 'alcopops', which were alcoholic sweet drinks in fashionable bottles. One of the first was called Hooch and advertised as 'wickedly refreshing'. However, its sweet lemonade taste and label design were criticised as being appealing to youngsters. At nearly 5 per cent proof it was relaunched with a more adult orientation. None the less, there were realistic fears about growing numbers of teenage binge drinkers in Britain.

Another growing trend was for body art and in particular henna tattoos, which had been popular in the 1960s. These wore off eventually and so were very popular as they did not incite the wrath of parents as much as permanent tattoos would have done. The singer Madonna in particular popularised them. However, real tattoos were also becoming increasingly popular, again with many 1990s pop, film and sports stars adopting them, such as Pamela Anderson and Johnny Depp. While they used to be used by film makers to portray rebellion, they were now coming to be seen as portraying individuality and 'cool'! 'Sporty Spice' was another ambassador, though she later grew to regret them. The Spice Girls were now very popular and their merchandising empire was in full swing with a range of Spice Girls dolls out just in time for Christmas. The toy store Hamley's even opened a special Spice Girls department.

Music

The success of the Spice Girls was mirrored at the Brit Awards where they won best single and video and performed *Wannabe* live with Geri Halliwell wearing that iconic Union Jack dress. Another teen band, Steps, were just emerging on their own journey to cult status, especially among schoolchildren. Their first hit song, *5,6,7,8*, had a line dancing routine to it and was one of the biggest-selling singles of the 1990s even though it never got into the top ten! The band Katrina and the Waves won the Eurovision Song Contest with the song *Love Shine a Light*, but the biggest song of the year was Elton John's reworked version of *Candle in the Wind* as a tribute to Diana, Princess of Wales. It became the second best-selling single ever, second only to Bing Crosby's *White Christmas*. Other hits this year included:

Barbie Girl	Aqua
Angels	Robbie Williams

I'll be Missing You	Puff Daddy and Faith Evans
D'You Know What I Mean?	Oasis
Tubthumping	Chumbawamba
Spice Up Your Life	Spice Girls
Teletubbies Say Eh-Oh!	Teletubbies
Men in Black	Will Smith
Don't Speak	No Doubt
Torn	Natalie Imbruglia

Television

This year saw the arrival of Po, Tinky Winky, Laa-Laa and Dipsy or the Teletubbies! These baby-faced, big-eared toddlers with antennae on their heads were clad in bright romper suits, spoke in gibberish and lived in Tellytubbyland. They played games and were supposed to appeal to infants. However, they caused some controversy by encouraging poor spoken English, for example saying 'eh-oh' instead of 'hello'. None the less they competed with the Spice Girls for the Christmas toy must-have spot. Another popular children's show doing well was *Power Rangers*, which also spawned a huge toy industry. Other debuts included *Jonathan Creek*, *Ally McBeal*, *Ground Force*, *Robot Wars*, *Midsomer Murders* and *I'm Alan Partridge*. In the world of adverts, we were treated to the funny spectacle of American bullfrogs calling to one another with the words 'bud' and 'weiser'!

Screen and page

Hollywood actor James Stewart died this year. He had a distinctive voice and played the archetypal good guy. Robert Mitchum also died this year and he was just the opposite, usually playing the archetypal tough guy. How many of their films can you name? Stewart's films included *It's a Wonderful Life*, *Harvey*, *The Philadelphia Story*, *Rear Window* and *How the West was Won*. Mitchum's included *Out of the Past*, *River of No Return*, *The Night of the Hunter*, *Cape Fear*, *Angel Face* and *Ryan's Daughter*.

Routledge
Taylor & Francis Group

Two of the best films released this year were *Titanic* and *The Full Monty*. *Titanic* starred Leonardo DiCaprio and Kate Winslet in a romantic epic tale of the disaster told via the love story of these two, one an Irish worker and the other a wealthy socialite. It cost over a billion dollars, had superb special effects and went on to win 11 Oscars. *The Full Monty* was a tale of unemployed Sheffield steel workers trying to make ends meet by turning themselves into a local version of the Chippendales. Starring Robert Carlyle and Tom Wilkinson, it had serious undertones about self-respect and dignity on the dole, but it was great fun too. In one memorable scene they lapse into their dance routine while waiting in the benefits queue. Made on a much lower budget than *Titanic*, it won the BAFTA for best film. This year also saw the 18th Bond film, *Tomorrow Never Dies*, with Pierce Brosnan as Bond and Jonathan Pryce as the villain.

Other films released this year included:

Austin Powers: International Man of Mystery	Mike Myers
Good Will Hunting	Robin Williams
Hercules	
L.A. Confidential	Kevin Spacey, Kim Basinger, Russell Crowe
The Lost World: Jurassic Park	Jeff Goldblum, Richard Attenborough
Men in Black	Will Smith, Tommy Lee Jones
The Devil's Advocate	Al Pacino, Keanu Reeves
Jackie Brown	Pam Grier

In literature, the year's publishing event was *Harry Potter and the Philosopher's Stone* by J. K. Rowling. This was to become cult reading and sell millions. Other books this year included *The Perfect Storm* by Sebastian Junger, Terry Pratchett's *Jingo*, Ian McEwan's *Enduring Love*, Bill Bryson's *A Walk in the Woods* and the poems *Tales from Ovid* by Ted Hughes.

Routledge
Taylor & Francis Group

Sport

It was a year of new homes in football! Sunderland's Stadium of Light, the largest football stadium to be built since the 1920s, was opened in July. Derby County moved into Pride Park, Bolton into the Reebok Stadium and Stoke City also moved into their new Britannia Stadium, which was opened by Sir Stanley Matthews. In golf, Tiger Woods rewrote the history book at the age of 21 when he won the US Masters. He was the youngest person to do so and the first black person. As well as this, his score beat the previous course record and he had the widest-ever winning margin. This was also the year the government announced that it was to ban sports sponsorship by tobacco firms, but it was to take until 2005 for this to become effective. It was also the year that the boxer Mike Tyson bit off part of Evander Holyfield's ear in a WBA Heavyweight Championship fight!

Do you remember?

1990s fashion fads! A fashion fad popular at this time was baseball caps, essential wear for rappers. These were often worn back to front by baseball players and this habit was adopted by many. Black-rimmed glasses were also back in vogue, with some, such as Chris Evans, trying to recreate the Michael Caine look, and were popularised by the film *Austin Powers, International Man of Mystery*. The 1990s also saw some dire hair trends, none more so than the 'rat's tail'! This was a long thin wisp of hair extending down a man's neck. Other fashion trends now considered bad mistakes were baggy shorts stopping midway between knee and ankle with lots of pockets in the legs, and a trend for wearing dungarees with just one shoulder done up. Others harked back to the 1960s and 1970s, with bandanas and crimped hair. The battle for the worst fashion decade is an open contest between the 1970s, 1980s and 1990s!

R Routledge Taylor & Francis Group

1997 Personal and local events

Routledge
Taylor & Francis Group

1998

Major events

January

The Monica Lewinsky scandal broke in the USA, with allegations of sexual and ethical misconduct by President Clinton. Clinton admitted to an inappropriate relationship with the White House intern, but the Senate later voted to acquit him.

March

Work started on the Millennium Dome on the Greenwich peninsula.

Rolls Royce was bought by BMW, the German car company.

April

The Good Friday Agreement was reached in Northern Ireland. A tentative agreement on the future of the peace process was worked out by Northern Ireland politicians after last-minute interventions by Tony Blair and Bill Clinton. The agreement made provisions for a Northern Ireland assembly with opposing factions sitting together to govern the province. Many fingers were crossed, hoping this would work out. David Trimble and John Hume were later awarded the Nobel Peace Prize for their role in the process.

May

Frank Sinatra died. Fans around the world mourned the death of the veteran crooner. His 1969 hit *My Way* became his signature tune and an all-time classic. In 1953 he won an Oscar for his role in the film *From Here to Eternity*.

June

The two pound coin was introduced.

July

Anti-Social Behaviour Orders (ASBOs) came into being.

August

Bomb attacks occurred on US embassies in Nairobi and Dar-es-Salaam. The attacks were linked to the Islamic fundamentalist Osama bin Laden.

A car bomb in Northern Ireland killed 29, making it the worst atrocity in the history of the Troubles.

September
David Trimble of the Ulster Unionist Party met with Gerry Adams of Sinn Fein, the first such meeting since 1922.

October
General Pinochet (82) was arrested on human rights charges. Lady Thatcher came to his support but legal proceedings began.

December
Storms lashed the country on Boxing Day.

Also this year ... Mohamed Al-Fayed claimed that there had been a conspiracy to kill his son and Princess Diana because of the scandal their relationship had brought to the state.

On the home front

The new car on the block was the Ford Focus, which was designed to take up the mantle of the successful Escort and was voted European car of the year. This was at a time when the term 'road rage' had just come into use. With ever-increasing numbers of cars on the roads, it was almost inevitable that congestion and rush hours would combine to test the patience of Britain's drivers. Most of it thankfully was confined to insults and hand gestures not in the highway code! One UK survey in the mid-1990s found that 60 per cent of us lost our temper behind the wheel and also resorted to practices such as tailgating and headlight flashing.

Meanwhile, younger people had found the perfect way to de-stress themselves and get revenge, the Super Soaker. These space age weapons had the ability to fire high-pressure jets of water long distances. A pump built up the water pressure in a tank and then the trigger unleashed it at a distant victim. Great fun! Over 250 million of them were made and bought by wary parents suspicious of their mischief potential!

Even younger people had no choice but to retire to the safety of their Little Tykes plastic log cabins or houses. The sturdy clip-together playhouses were very popular in the 1990s and made great ready-built dens.

Routledge Taylor & Francis Group

Things were changing in the world of food, too. The Food Standards Agency found that it took an hour to prepare a meal in 1980 but just 20 minutes by 1990. Chicken tikka masala was well on the way to being declared the nation's favourite dish, while for breakfast Pop Tarts were in vogue. These were thin sheets of pastry with a sweet filling which you just popped in the toaster. In the world of sweets, old favourites were still high on the list, the decade's best sellers being Kit Kats, Mars Bars, Cadbury's Dairy Milk and Roses. The only non-chocolate item in the top ten was Wrigley's chewing gum. Newer fads included fizzy crystals such as Fizz Whizz, which popped and fizzed on your tongue, Push Pops, the sticky lollipops in lipstick-like plastic tubes, bubble gum tape in a roll and very long Sherbert Straws.

Music

The year's best hits included:

Believe	Cher
My Heart Will Go On	Celine Dion
It's Like That	Run-DMC vs Jason Nevins
No Matter What	Boyzone
C'est la Vie	B*Witched
Millennium	Robbie Williams
Dance the Night Away	The Mavericks
I Don't Want to Miss a Thing	Aerosmith
Heartbeat	Steps

Veteran crooner Frank Sinatra died this year. He was also a film star, but can you recall some of his greatest hits? They included *High Hopes*, *My Kind of Town*, *Strangers in the Night*, *I've Got You Under My Skin*, *You Make Me Feel So Young* and *My Way*.

Routledge
Taylor & Francis Group

Television

Shock horror, the BBC *Blue Peter* presenter Richard Bacon was sacked after a *News of the World* report alleged he took cocaine. Televison debuts included *The Royle Family, Scrapheap Challenge, Bob the Builder* and *Who Wants to be a Millionaire? 'Millionaire'*, as it became known, was presented by Chris Tarrant and contestants had to answer 15 (later 12) questions to win £1 million. They had three lifelines to help them: 'ask the audience', '50/50' and 'phone a friend'.

Screen and page

This year's best films included:

The Big Lebowski	Jeff Bridges, John Goodman
Saving Private Ryan	Tom Hanks
A Bug's Life	
Armageddon	Bruce Willis
Mulan	
Shakespeare In Love	Gwyneth Paltrow, Joseph Fiennes
Rush Hour	Jackie Chan, Chris Tucker
Small Soldiers	Kirsten Dunst
You've Got Mail	Tom Hanks, Meg Ryan

Poet Ted Hughes died this year. He was an 'earthy' and distinctive poet with a gift for portraying the natural world in an unsentimental way. He had a troubled relationship with his wife, the poet Sylvia Plath, who committed suicide in 1963. Poet Laureate for 14 years, this year also saw the publication of his book *Birthday Letters* just months before he died. His other works included *Hawk in the Rain, Lupercal, Wodwo* and *Crow*. He was also the author of children's stories including *The Iron Man*.

Other books published this year were *Harry Potter and the Chamber of Secrets* by J. K. Rowling, *About a Boy* by Nick Hornby, *The No 1 Ladies Detective Agency* by Alexander McCall Smith, Ian McEwan's *Amsterdam* and *England, England* by Julian Barnes.

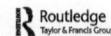

Sport

This year saw the Winter Olympics in Nagano, Japan. Great Britain's only medal was a bronze in the four-man bobsleigh. In contrast to this, at the European Athletics Championships in Budapest GB ended at the top of the medals table, with the men taking the 100, 200, 400, 4×100 and 4×400 metres titles. Jonathan Edwards won the triple jump and Steve Backley the javelin, while Denise Lewis took the women's heptathlon. This was also World Cup year, hosted by France who went on to beat Brazil 3–0 in the final at the Stade de France. Zinedine Zidane scored twice for France with Emmanuel Petit adding the third. England meanwhile had a strong team and were unlucky not to reach the quarter-finals and beyond. They were knocked out by Argentina who, after a score of 2–2 at full time, went on to win on penalties. David Beckham was red-carded in this game for kicking out at an opponent who had fouled him. Had he stayed on and taken a penalty … who knows? Alan Shearer and Michael Owen both scored their penalties and were England's top scorers in the tournament with two goals apiece.

Do you remember?

Girls' and music magazines. The best-selling teenage girls' magazines in 1998 were *Smash Hits*, *Just 17*, *Looks*, *Jackie*, *Mizz*, *Company*, *19*, *Number One*, *Girl*, *Blue Jeans* and *My Guy*. In the early 1990s young teenage girls all wanted to read about Kylie, Jason and boy bands, but later they were becoming more fashion conscious and so adult women's magazines such as *Vogue*, *Cosmopolitan* and *Elle* brought out teenage versions. Many girls' magazines revolved around readers' stories and embarrassments and celebrity gossip, articles about dating strategies and quizzes about pop stars, and of course the secrets of being a great kisser! Some producers changed their target audience to what were called 'tweenagers', the nine to 13 age group, with titles such as *It's HOT*. In music, the BBC brought out *Top of the Pops* magazine and readers were turning away from the older newspaper-style *Melody Maker* and *New Musical Express*. Glossy magazines were the way forward. In 1998 even these magazines were struggling to compete with digital and online media, so much had the world changed!

1998 Personal and local events

Routledge
Taylor & Francis Group

1999

Major events

January

The Euro was launched. It was adopted by 11 countries initially, but Euro notes and coins would not come in until 2002 with the old coinage being gradually phased out. Can you remember what the currency of these 'Euro' countries used to be? Spain: Peseta, Germany: Mark, Greece: Drachma, Italy: Lira, The Netherlands: Guilder and Portugal: Escudo.

Prince Edward became engaged to Sophie Rhys-Jones.

February

King Hussein of Jordan died; he had ruled Jordan for 46 years.

March

NATO launched air strikes against Yugoslavia. Tensions rose in Kosovo between Serbian forces under President Slobodan Milosevic and the majority ethnic Albanian population. The Serbs had been guilty of massacres of ethnic Albanian civilians and driving tens of thousands of them out of their homes in a campaign of 'ethnic cleansing'.

A Mont Blanc tunnel fire killed 40.

April

A minimum wage of £3.60 an hour was set for the over-21s.

Television presenter Jill Dando was shot dead on her doorstep.

May

The Scottish Parliament met for the first time, as did the Welsh Assembly.

Princess Anne opened the Midland Metro, a tram system between Birmingham and Wolverhampton which ran along old railway lines.

June

Prince Edward married Sophie Rhys-Jones.

Routledge
Taylor & Francis Group

July

Neil Kinnock was appointed vice-president of the European Commission.

August

Charles Kennedy became leader of the Liberal Democrats.

A spectacular total solar eclipse was watched by millions in Europe.

Tony Martin, a Norfolk farmer, was charged with the murder of a burglar he shot dead in his home. This case sparked a great debate about our rights to defend ourselves in our own homes.

October

Two trains collided at Ladbroke Grove junction near Paddington, killing 31. The trial of GP murderer Harold Shipman began. He was accused of killing 15 patients between 1995 and 1998.

The London Eye big wheel was set into position on the South Bank.

December

George Harrison, the former Beatle, was stabbed by an intruder at his home.

Midnight sparked huge Millennium celebrations across the world.

Also this year ... unemployment fell to below 1.3 million, the lowest for 20 years, and artist Tracey Emin exhibited *My Bed* at the Tate Gallery. It was 'as slept in', with cigarette ends, empty drinks bottles and dirty underwear. It sold for £150,000.

On the home front

Our infatuation with celebrity was well catered for this year with the celebrity weddings of Victoria 'Posh Spice' Adams and David Beckham, and Zoe Ball and the DJ Fat Boy Slim. The Beckhams were paid a huge sum to allow *OK* magazine to have a world exclusive at the wedding ... 'the pictures the world has waited to see'! The paparazzi photographers would have been trying hard to sneak some unofficial snaps of this event. They may well have been fortified in their efforts by one of the many energy drinks coming on to the market, such as Red Bull. The slogan for this

Routledge
Taylor & Francis Group

told you 'it gives you wings'! Containing caffeine, many young people used it to help them party all night in clubs. Another emerging craze was texting on mobile phones and this cheap method of communication was soon wholeheartedly embraced by the young. Many shorthand terms and abbreviations have emerged, such as just using 'U' instead of 'you', much to the annoyance of teachers, who sometimes feel that it stops children learning to spell correctly.

Do you know what these mean?

2MO	*tomorrow*
4eva	*forever*
BFN	*bye for now*
BLNT	*better luck next time*
CUL8R	*see you later*
GR8	*great*
IU2U	*it's up to you*
K	*okay*
LOL	*laughing out loud*
OMG	*oh my God*
ORLY	*oh really*
I<3 U	*I love you*

Music

Boy bands were still very much at the height of popularity. Boyzone, with Ronan Keating and Stephen Gately, had two chart-topping hits including *When The Going Gets Tough*. They split up and Keating went on to have a huge solo hit with *When You Say Nothing At All*. The biggest act, however, were Westlife, whose first four singles including *I Have a Dream* went straight to number one. Meanwhile, two girls were fighting for supremacy: Britney Spears and Christina Aguilera both released their first singles *Baby One More Time* and *Genie in a Bottle* and both went to number one. Rap and Garage music were also doing well again with the likes of Eminem coming on the scene. Other hits this year included:

Livin La Vida Loca	Ricky Martin
Mambo No 5 (A Little Bit of…)	Lou Bega
Blue (Da Ba Dee)	Eiffel 65
The Millennium Prayer	Cliff Richard
That Don't Impress Me Much	Shania Twain
Bring It All Back	S Club 7

This year saw the death of Dusty Springfield, aged 59, after a battle with breast cancer. Her songs included *You Don't Have To Say You Love Me, I Just Don't Know What To Do With Myself* and the classic *I Only Want To be With You.*

Yehudi Menuhin, the virtuoso violinist, also died this year aged 83. He gave his first concert at the age of seven and is remembered by many for his collaborations with jazz violinist Stephane Grappelli.

Television

Two successful blockbusters came to the small screen this year. *Sex in the City* starred Sarah Jessica Parker and Kim Catterall as New York singles. It revolved around a group of four friends and their sexual adventures. On a more serious note, *Walking with Dinosaurs* was a superb documentary using computer-generated images of dinosaurs which explored how they might have lived and died. This year also saw the debut of Jamie Oliver's *Naked Chef* cookery programme. With his cheeky 'laddish' style and Essex accent he took a relaxed approach to cooking. Also debuting was the *11 O'Clock Show*, which took a satirical look at the world and introduced Sacha Baron Cohen as his alter ego Ali G. He played a white British male with strong stereotypical views who was into Jamaican and Rap culture. He interviewed celebrities and politicians, asking very naive questions and often getting them to say things they regretted. Other debuts included *Holby City, Grand Designs* and *Bremner, Bird and Fortune.* The face of BBC sport also changed radically this year when Des Lynam left the BBC. *Match of the Day* would never be the same but he was ably succeeded by Gary Lineker.

Routledge Taylor & Francis Group

Screen and page

Perhaps this year's most popular film was *The Matrix*. The plot is that we are living in a simulated world called the Matrix which is run by computers who use our body heat as a source of energy! The hero Neo, played by Keanu Reeves, rebels against this regime. The film used very good slow motion special effects. The scariest film of the year was *The Blair Witch Project*, where three students go missing, leaving behind only the documentary film they were making about a local witch legend. Other good films included:

American Beauty	Kevin Spacey
Star Wars: Episode I – The Phantom Menace	Ewan McGregor, Liam Neeson
The Mummy	Brendan Fraser, Rachel Weiss
Fight Club	Brad Pitt
The Green Mile	Tom Hanks
Sleepy Hollow	Johnny Depp
Notting Hill	Hugh Grant
Eyes Wide Shut	Nicole Kidman, Tom Cruise
The World Is Not Enough	Pierce Brosnan

Hell-raising actor Oliver Reed died this year; his films included *Oliver*, *Women in Love*, *The Devils* and *The Three Musketeers*. Dirk Bogarde also died, leaving behind a huge legacy of films including *The Blue Lamp*, *The Sea Shall Not Have Them*, *Doctor In The House*, *Death in Venice* and *The Night Porter*.

In literature, the year's best books included J. K. Rowling's *Harry Potter and the Prisoner of Azkaban*, J. M. Coetzee's *Disgrace*, *Girl with a Pearl Earring* by Tracy Chevalier, *The Bad Beginning (A Series of Unfortunate Events)* by Lemony Snicket, *The Amber Spyglass* by Philip Pullman and *Chocolat* by Joanne Harris.

Sport

In football, England manager Glenn Hoddle was sacked in February following comments he made suggesting that the disabled were being punished for sins in a previous life. He was replaced by Kevin Keegan. The Geordie Bobby Robson became Newcastle manager, much to the home fans' delight. But the footballing event of the year was Manchester United beating Bayern Munich 2–1 in the Champions League final. After the match United manager Alex Ferguson gave his oft-quoted summary of the game, 'Football; bloody hell'. This victory gave United the treble as they had already won the Premiership and FA Cup. Ferguson was later knighted for his services to football. The 16 October this year proved a dismal day for football as a total of 26 players were sent off in the Football League, the biggest number of dismissals in its history!

In rugby, the Millennium Stadium in Cardiff was opened but Scotland won the last ever Five Nations Championship. From 2000 it was to be Six Nations, with Italy joining the fray.

Do you remember?

Pokemon! This started out as a Nintendo Game Boy video game and developed into a cult card game. Coming from Japan, it became a massive craze with children spending all their pocket money on the cards in the late 1990s. Pokemon is short for pocket monsters and each card has a creature with special skills. In the video game a boy has to capture and train Pokemon, whose names included Pikachu, Squirtle, Beedrill, Pidgeotto and Jigglypuff. It all sounded a bit Tellytubbies, but to millions of children it was very serious. It spawned even more electronic games and several films. A television series had a young boy, Ash, and his two friends Misty and Brock searching the world for other Pokemon. Game players collect and train Pokemon and try to reach the level of Pokemon Master. You capture other Pokemon by throwing a Pokeball at them and trainers can send their Pokemon to battle others. This was the idea behind the card game where each Pokemon card had certain strengths and values which could be enhanced by the use of special energy cards.

Routledge
Taylor & Francis Group

1999 Personal and local events

Routledge
Taylor & Francis Group

2000

Major events

January

As the Millennium celebrations continued, the Queen opened the Millennium Dome. Fears of major collapses in computers because of the date change for the Millennium proved to be unfounded. Nothing happened!

Dr Harold Shipman was sentenced to life imprisonment.

February

The Royal Bank of Scotland took over NatWest.

March

General Pinochet was returned to Chile to face trial.

April

Norfolk farmer Tony Martin was given a life sentence for the murder of the 16-year-old burglar he shot in his home. The sentence was eventually reduced to manslaughter and he served three years.

May

May Day riots in London by anti-capitalist protestors saw a statue of Churchill daubed with paint and slogans.

Ken Livingstone was elected as Mayor of London on 4 May. The day is also significant for *Star Wars* fans … May the fourth (be with you)!

Vladimir Putin was inaugurated as President of Russia after the resignation of Boris Yeltsin the previous year.

Two Royal Marines, Alan Chambers and Charlie Paton, became the first men to reach the North Pole unaided.

June

The Millennium Bridge in London opened but had to be closed after it started swaying.

Routledge
Taylor & Francis Group

July

An Air France Concorde jet crashed, killing all 100 passengers and nine crew.

August

The Queen Mother celebrated her 100th birthday.

September

There were large fuel protests, with lorry drivers blocking refineries in protest at high fuel prices. This led to panic buying and a petrol shortage when garages ran out.

October

Wembley Stadium closed after 77 years. It was to be completely reconstructed to seat more people. The famous twin towers were demolished.

A GNER InterCity 225 derailed at high speed just outside Hatfield, killing four people.

November

Michael Douglas married Catherine Zeta-Jones.

Ten-year-old schoolboy Damilola Taylor was stabbed to death on his way home from school.

December

Heavy snow and temperatures as low as minus 13 brought havoc to travel and as the year closed it was recorded as the wettest year ever for the UK.

Also this year ... Judith Keppel became the first person to win a million on *Who Wants to be a Millionaire?* In reality there was still a wide rich–poor divide, with figures showing that average spending on food was just £26 a week for the poorest tenth of households and £111 for the richest. The Queen opened the Tate Modern gallery in May. It was housed in the transformed Bankside Power Station and quickly became a respected international venue for contemporary art.

Routledge
Taylor & Francis Group

On the home front

By 2000 the UK population had reached nearly 60 million, with 20 per cent under the age of 16 and 7 per cent describing themselves as belonging to an ethnic minority, reflecting the increasingly multicultural nature of Britain. This was backed up by a survey of our eating habits and sales of chilled foods which found that roughly a quarter of meals were Italian and a quarter Indian, with only about 20 per cent traditional British meals.

In 2000 cohabitation was more common and around 20 per cent of births were to cohabiting couples. Marriage rates had been dropping since the 1970s and marriage had become less of an economic necessity as many women had paid work outside the home. Alongside this people were marrying later, with working women postponing marriage in favour of establishing a career. Divorce had also become more common after the 1969 Divorce Reform Act. This had introduced the 'no fault' divorce and helped reduce some of the stigma attached to it, so that by 2000 around 40 per cent of marriages would break down. Alongside this was an increasing number of people being lone parents. For those who did have children, the most popular babies' names of 2000 were Chloe, Emily and Megan for girls and Jack, Thomas and James for boys. Chloe and Jack were not even in the top 100 in the early 1970s, when the top names were Michael and Jennifer. Sixty per cent of the population regarded themselves as belonging to a religion (55 per cent were Christian), though on many census forms quite a few put their religion down as Jedi! Politically, people were becoming a little jaded and in the 2001 general election the turnout was just 59 per cent, the lowest since 1918, with those under 34 being the least likely to vote. The most popular national newspaper was the *Sun* with the *Telegraph* and *Times* being the most popular broadsheets.

This was the year that saw micro-scooters rival skateboards for the Christmas toy market. They were very popular and some adults even used them for their commute to work … but not for long. Pokemon was still a huge craze, while Bob the Builder merchandise kept the younger ones pleased. The best-selling game of the year was a board game version of *Who Wants to be a Millionaire?*

Home entertainment was a growth area, with 4.5 million households having satellite or cable television, but at the same time cinema attendance doubled between 1984 and 2000 with the growth of multiplex cinemas. Nearly 50 per cent of households had a mobile phone and 45 per cent a computer. Ninety-three per cent of us had a washing

R Routledge
Taylor & Francis Group

machine compared with 65 per cent in 1970, and many other labour-saving devices had become more common. By far the biggest pastime was watching television, closely followed by entertaining friends and listening to the radio and music. Since the early 1990s the choice of television channels had grown enormously, as had the sales of videos. The best-selling video of 2000 was *Toy Story 2* and the most rented was *The Sixth Sense.* DVDs were becoming the fastest-growing format and would soon render the video obsolete, as CDs generally did to vinyl records. Around 58 per cent of males and 70 per cent of females read books regularly, but library use was in serious decline. Gardening and DIY were more popular with the middle-aged. Seventy-two per cent of us gambled regularly, mainly on the National Lottery. Six and a half million visited the Millennium Experience, making it the most popular day attraction. The most popular European holiday destination was still Spain.

In sport, football was the most popular activity for boys and swimming for girls. Overall, the most common physical activity was walking, though for most this was not very far and not very often. Around 15 per cent of all children were obese, as were around 21 per cent of adults, and these figures were set to rise yearly, with many lamenting the reduced amount of time children spent doing PE in school and the growth in fast food outlets and sedentary electronic pastimes. The couch potato was still much in evidence, though maybe more of a computer potato!

Music

British acts were dominating the charts, with U2 back on form with the album *All That You Can't Leave Behind* and the Coldplay debut *Parachutes.* Kylie was back to number one with *Spinning Around* and the Beatles ended the year on top of the album charts with a greatest hits release called *1*; it became the fastest-selling album of all time. The Christmas number one was *Can We Fix It* by Bob the Builder!

This year's other hits included:

Rock DJ	Robbie Williams
Oops! ... I Did It Again	Britney Spears
Pure Shores	All Saints
Stan	Eminem

Routledge
Taylor & Francis Group

Who Let The Dogs Out	Baha Men
Groovejet (If This Ain't Love)	Spiller featuring Sophie Ellis Bextor
Beautiful Day	U2

Television

BBC News went to 10pm, upsetting those who had got used to the nine o'clock slot. But the big event was the debut of *Big Brother*. This was either an interesting study in group living or (more likely) a confirmation of our obsession with celebrities and voyeurism. Other debuts this year included *Castaway*, *Monarch of the Glen* and *The Weakest Link*. As contestants voted each other off, host Anne Robinson would utter the humiliating phrase, 'You are the weakest link. Goodbye!'

Screen and page

This year's top movies included:

Gladiator	Russell Crowe
The Beach	Leonardo DiCaprio
American Psycho	Christian Bale
Castaway	Tom Hanks
Chocolat	Juliette Binoche, Johnny Depp
Crouching Tiger, Hidden Dragon	Yun-Fat Chow
The Perfect Storm	George Clooney
Billy Elliot	Jamie Bell
Chicken Run	

The English actor Alec Guinness died this year. He made over 55 films, many of them classics, including *Great Expectations, Kind Hearts and Coronets* (where he played eight roles!), *The Bridge On The River Kwai* and *Star Wars*, and the television dramatisation of *Tinker, Tailor, Soldier, Spy*.

In literature, the year's popular books included J. K. Rowling's *Harry Potter and the Goblet of Fire*, Dan Brown's *Angels and Demons*, Margaret Atwood's *The Blind Assassin* and *White Teeth* by Zadie Smith.

Sport

Chelsea beat Aston Villa 1–0 in the last FA Cup Final at Wembley Stadium before it was rebuilt. The last England match in the old stadium was, would you believe it, a 1–0 defeat to Germany. The match was captain Tony Adams' 60th appearance there, which was a record, and he was also the last Englishman to score there. Manager Kevin Keegan resigned after this game to be replaced by Sven-Goran Eriksson, the first foreign manager to take charge of the England team. In the UEFA Cup Arsenal lost to Galatasaray on penalties after a 0–0 draw. It was the first time a Turkish team had won a European title. In cycling, the legendary Lance Armstrong won the Tour de France for the second time. He was to go on to win it seven consecutive times in all, only to be stripped of all of these titles in 2012 for drug offences. In golf, Tiger Woods won the British Open, the US Open and the PGA Championship. In the Sydney Olympics, Britons won 11 gold medals, including Jonathan Edwards in the triple jump, Audley Harrison in boxing, Denise Lewis in the heptathlon, Ben Ainslie in sailing and Steve Redgrave winning his fifth gold in the men's coxless fours. At Wimbledon, Venus Williams won the ladies' singles and the women's doubles with her sister Serena. She was to go on to win both four more times! And in rugby union, England won the first-ever Six Nations Championship.

Do you remember?

Television ads and celebrity catchphrases! Can you remember these

Maybe, just maybe	*National Lottery*
Do it before you …	*Chewit*
Doh!	*Homer Simpson*
Impossible is nothing	*Adidas*
I don't believe it	*Victor Meldrew*

Hasta la vista baby	*Terminator*
Is that your final answer?	*Who Wants to be a Millionaire?*
How will you eat yours?	*Cadbury Creme Egg*
Coffee at its best	*Nescafé*
Because you're worth it	*L'Oreal*
Melts in your mouth not in your hands	*M&Ms*
The car in front is a …	*Toyota*
Higher! Lower!	*Play Your Cards Right*
Maybe she's born with it, maybe it's …	*Maybelline*
Get busy with the fizzy	*SodaStream*
Everything we do is driven by you	*Ford*
Nothing else quite hits the mark	*Strongbow Cider*
Small ones are more juicy	*Outspan oranges*
The card that puts you in charge	*American Express*
To infinity and beyond	*Buzz Lightyear*

2000 Personal and local events

Routledge
Taylor & Francis Group